Critical Reading for the Reflective Practitioner

A Guide for Primary Care

Health Learning Center

Department of Nursing Development
251 E. Huron
Chicago, IL 60611

NM **Northwestern Memorial Hospital**

This book is dedicated to our families

Critical Reading for the Reflective Practitioner

A Guide for Primary Care

Robert Clarke

General Practitioner, Potters Bar and Associate Dean,
Department of Postgraduate General Practice, North Thames (West),
Imperial College School of Medicine, London, UK

Peter Croft

Department of Epidemiology, University of Keele, UK

Forword by
Professor Patrick Pietroni

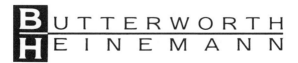

OXFORD   AUCKLAND   BOSTON   JOHANNESBURG   MELBOURNE   NEW DELHI

Butterworth-Heinemann
Linacre House, Jordan Hill, Oxford OX2 8DP
225 Wildwood Avenue, Woburn, MA 01801–2041
A division of Reed Educational and Professional Publishing Ltd

A member of the Reed Elsevier plc group

First published 1998

British Library Cataloguing in Publication Data
A catalogue record for this book is available from the British Library

Library of Congress Cataloguing in Publication Data
A catalogue record for this book is available from the Library of
Congress

ISBN 0 7506 3939 3

Composition by Genesis Typesetting, Laser Quay, Rochester, Kent
Printed and bound in Great Britain by
Biddles Ltd, Guildford and King's Lynn

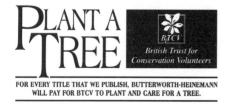

Contents

Foreword

It is rare to read a book which is both timely and ahead of its time. With the Health Service reforms accelerating as a consequence of the new Government – the ability to reflect, and more importantly to reflect critically, has become an essential ingredient for the future clinician.

The new language of managed health care and evidence-based medicine is rapidly entering the field of Primary Care. Practitioners will increasingly be asked to account both clinically and financially for the decisions they make in their consulting rooms. Patients, although better informed, are also more confused as conflicting advice on health promotion, food safety and surgical procedures multiplies.

The 'scientific-method' has stood the test of time for many disciplines and is the foundation for much of modern medicine. In the last two decades this approach to the study of human health and disease has been found limiting – especially in primary care. The concepts of reflective practice and critical enquiry build on the strengths of the scientific method but take it into the 'swampy lowlands' of General Practice.

Dr Clarke and Professor Croft have provided an essential text to these developments in the way we think and the way we work. They write in an easily readable, creative and entertaining style – demonstrating the art of reflective practice and critical reading in the manner in which this important book is presented. I predict this book will become an essential *vade mecum* for all practitioners.

Professor Patrick C. Pietroni
Dean of Postgraduate General Practice
North Thames (West)

Acknowledgements

We wish to thank the many colleagues and friends who have supported us in writing this book. In particular, we thank the patients, staff and partners of Highview Medical Centre, Potters Bar for their encouragement. We also acknowledge the help of all those who have attended the Barnet Critical Reading Course where many of our ideas have been developed. We owe a lot to the Royal College of General Practitioners who in 1990 introduced a specific paper on critical reading into the Membership examination. This not only set an appropriate agenda for general practitioners but also provided us with some excellent examples for discussion, many of which are used in this book. We would also like to thank Guy Robinson, Mary Davies and Tom Roper of the Barnet Postgraduate Centre Library and Information Service for all the support they have provided, without which none of this would have been possible. Adrian Barnes and Chris McManus inspired one of us (RC) to overcome his fear of numbers and look for the ideas behind basic statistics. Geoff Smaldon, of Butterworth-Heinemann, has been extremely encouraging from the beginning and his patience knows no bounds.

Tom Boyd was the person who suggested that we write this book and we hold him entirely responsible for all the time we have spent away from our families. Many others have read and commented on parts or all of the manuscript. These include:

Ann and Alan Clarke, Roslynne Freeman, Andrew Gellert, Chris Jenner, Geoff Hackett, Felicity Light, Hugh Mather, Roger Neighbour, Patrick Pietroni, Roger Pietroni, Martin Roland, Andrew Wilson, Robert Winter, Paquita de Zuluetta.

We are grateful not only to these but to all who have made helpful comments about our approach to critical reading.

We would also like to thank the authors of all the texts from which we have quoted or which form the basis of our examples. They were bold enough actually to do the research and so stimulated our reading and reflection.

The authors and publishers would like to thank the following for permission to reproduce material in this book: Feder, G., Griffiths, C., Highton, C., Eldridge, S., Spence, M., and Southgate, L. (1995) Do clinical guidelines introduced with practice based education improve care of asthmatic and diabetic patients? A randomised controlled trial in general practice in East London. *British Medical Journal*, **311**, 1473–1478; Gillam, S.J. (1991) Understanding the uptake of cervical cancer screening: the contribution of the health belief model. [Review]. *British Journal of General Practice*, **41**, 510–513; Greenhalgh, P. (1994) Shared care for diabetes: a systematic review. Occasional paper 67 edn, 1–35. London: Royal College of General Practitioners; Jones, K., Charlton, I., Middleton, M., Preece, W., and Hill, A. (1992) Targeting asthma care in general practice using a morbidity index. *British Medical Journal*, **304**, 1353–1356; Jones, R. (1992) Decision making and hospital referrals. In: *Hospital Referrals* (Roland, M. and Coulter, A., eds), pp. 92–106. Oxford: Oxford University Press; Jones, R. and Kinmonth, A. (1995) *Critical Reading For Primary Care*. Oxford: Oxford University Press; Keeley, D. (1993) How to achieve better outcome in treatment of asthma in general practice. *British Medical Journal*, **307**, 1261–1263; Mathers, N. and Gask, L. (1995) Surviving the 'heartsink' experience. *Family Practice*, **12**, 176–183; Norton, K., and Smith, S. (1994) *Problems with Patients: Managing Complicated Transactions*. Cambridge: Cambridge University Press; Sackett, D., Richardson, W. and Haynes, R. (1997) *Evidence-based Medicine: How to Practise and Teach EBM*. London: Churchill Livingstone; Silverman, J., Kurtz, S., and Draper, J. (1996) The Calgary–Cambridge approach to communication skills teaching 1: agenda-led outcome-based analysis of the consultation. *Education for General Practice*, **7**, 288–299; Stoate, H.G. (1989) Can health screening damage your health? *Journal of the Royal College of General Practitioners*, **39**, 193–195. The Diabetes Control and Complications Trial Research Group (1993) The effect of intensive treatment of diabetes on the development of long-term complications in insulin-dependent diabetes mellitus. *New England Journal of Medicine*, **329**, 977–986.

R Clarke
P Croft

Introduction

'Evidence-based medicine' (EBM) has become a catchphrase of the 1990s. It carries a clear message: that reading, interpreting and acting on published literature should become a routine part of clinical practice. A fine ideal, perhaps, but it sounds like a full-time job in itself.

The dilemma is simple. To be a statistician or an epidemiologist or a social scientist demands a detailed knowledge of the subject, its concepts and its methods – the technical apparatus looks formidable. Any attempt to take on board all the fine detail which goes into the research endeavour is to court boredom at best, frustration at least, panic and mental anaesthesia at worst. How much of this knowledge does the busy and interested primary care practitioner need in order to assess the results of research?

Our view is that detail matters less than the understanding of the main ideas and central concepts. Much of the interpretation of a piece of research is to do with the broad knowledge which all practitioners can bring to a topic. This common sense approach sometimes seems to be missing from research papers remote from the daily practicalities of dealing with actual patients.

This book sets out to provide a logical structure which can channel common sense and practical experience into a formal evaluation and interpretation of published work.

We make a basic distinction between two labels, critical appraisal and critical reflection which refer to the two aspects of critical reading which we address in this book.

Critical reading

Two main components:

- Critical appraisal;
- Critical reflection.

CRITICAL APPRAISAL

Critical appraisal involves the assessment of the science and the quality of the study under scrutiny, its design, methods and analysis. This is the aspect which draws on methodological and statistical concepts. In this book we have tried to focus on how such concepts can be used and applied without getting bogged down in the detail and with minimal use of technical language. We have incorporated explanations of unavoidable terms in jargon corner boxes.

Jargon corner

Critical appraisal

Assessment of the scientific quality of a paper, including design, methods and analysis.

REFLECTION AND REFLECTIVE PRACTICE

The terms reflection and reflective practice are increasingly used in primary care and can have a number of different meanings:

- the ability to stand back and look at the way you practice;
- the ability to relate theory to practice;
- the ability to consider the broader context in which you work including organizational, social, ideological and political aspects;
- the ability to challenge implicit assumptions which frame working practices;
- the ability to reflect on yourself; your feelings as well as your thoughts and actions.

Reflective practice has the broad meaning of looking at your own professional behaviour with the intention of improving and developing. The process of reflection can involve thinking, reading and writing, discussion, use of audio and video, as well as role play. The term reflection is often used in a broad way to include these different levels of meaning and we have no problem with this inclusive use.

Some authors find it helpful to be more specific in defining exactly which aspect is being used. For example, a recent model of higher education discusses three domains to which criticality might apply; knowledge, self and the world. Matching each of these are critical reasoning, critical self-reflection and critical action (Barnett, 1997).

At different points in the text we invite the reader to pause and reflect (with reflection stop boxes) and we hope that a broad range

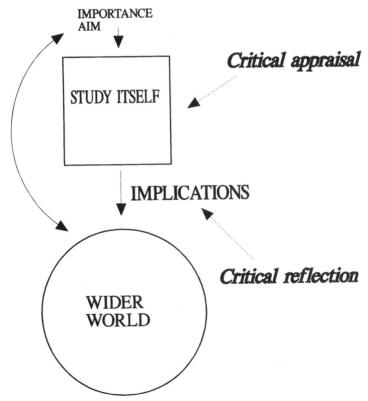

Figure 1. A study in context; critical appraisal and critical reflection.

of relevant thoughts, feelings and insights will result. However there is a narrow sense in which reflection can be used to relate the findings of research to actual practice and we use the term 'critical reflection' to describe this (Fig. 1).

CRITICAL REFLECTION

Critical reflection covers the systematic ways in which knowledge and experience can be used to judge the implications and applications of a published study. This aspect of critical reading often seems to be neglected in the evidence-based medicine philosophy. We believe that the only way to bring critical reading down from the ivory tower and into the market place is to give critical reflection techniques equal weight to those of critical appraisal.

Jargon corner

Critical reflection

Using a practitioner's knowledge and experience to relate research findings to practice.

WHAT DO WE MEAN BY CRITICAL APPRAISAL IN THIS BOOK?

Even if you do not wish to be a statistician or a researcher yourself, it can be useful to be able to judge some simple but essential aspects of how well a piece of research has been done.

Many practitioners doubt their ability to make such judgements. If you are one of them, try to answer two short questions.

Question stop

An opinion poll was carried out 1 week before the general election. A sample of people was stopped as they left Conservative Clubs in a number of different parts of the country, and they were asked how they intended to vote the following week. Ninety per cent said they would vote Conservative. 'Looks like we're heading for a landslide' said a beaming Tory.

What is the problem with his conclusion?

Comment

We are sure you can spot what is wrong with this. It is a completely hopeless sample for judging the voting intentions of the country as a whole. Being able to identify that means you are a critical appraiser: you can spot the big flaw.

Question stop

An opinion poll was carried out 1 week before the general election. A careful random selection was made from all people aged 18 and above in the United Kingdom. There were 10 people in the sample. Eight said they would vote Conservative. 'Looks like we're heading for a landslide,' said a beaming Tory.

What is the problem with his conclusion?

Comment

Again we think that you will spot what is wrong with the statement. It's too small a sample, however beautifully constructed, to say anything about the huge sample of the population who will be voting the subsequent week. So you're a statistician too, and have a feeling for the vagaries of chance.

This is basically what we mean by critical appraisal: a set of accessible skills, mostly logical, but some numerate, which allow you to examine systematically, but in not too much detail, the way in which a study has been done.

There is a growing science of systematic reviewing, in which groups of individuals collaborate to review a topic formally, using a structured format and analysis. The Cochrane Collaboration is the foremost international forum for such systematic reviewing. This text is not designed for the reader who is involved in such activities. This is an introduction to more general, day-to-day appraisal for those who have not tried it before or who want to extend their basic skills. We believe that only a few of these are needed to enable you to make sense of published papers and extract the take-home messages for your own practice.

WHAT DO WE MEAN BY REFLECTION AND CRITICAL REFLECTION IN THIS BOOK?

In 'pure science' conditions are carefully controlled so that the effect of one or two variables can be studied. This is epitomized in medical science by the randomized controlled trial which is regarded as the gold standard of EBM.

The reality of working in primary care is frequently quite unlike the situation of a randomized controlled trial. Although many of the problems presented by patients are in areas where evidence exists, each patient is unique and the approach of the generalist is to consider in a holistic way the physical, psychological and social influences which contribute to the presentation. We may be aware of previous problems for individuals and of the family, community and social context of their lives. At first glance, this can all seem miles away from a randomized controlled trial.

EBM quite rightly emphasizes the skills involved in forming a specific answerable question from a problem in practice. This includes selecting just part of the presentation for analysis, and necessarily implies that a large part will be left out. At worst this is the type of process whereby patients are categorized as 'a case of . . .' rather than as a human being living in the real world who is suffering from a particular set of problems. Because of this process of removing the context, EBM can seem to be obsessed with detail and unable to see the whole picture.

It is the whole picture which is of most concern to the practitioner. This can involve contact with dirty reality, with what Schon called the 'swampy lowlands'. This context is characterized by complexity, instability, constant change, the uniqueness of individual patients, uncertainty, and the ethical problems and value conflicts of dealing with people's everyday problems (Schon, 1983). The danger of EBM is that the context gets ignored.

Jargon corner

The swampy lowlands of primary care

Reality of working in primary care involves a complex context which is often simplified in clinical trials. Uncertainty, instability, the uniqueness of each individual and ethical issues affect the process of care. Evidence-based medicine needs to take these into account.

The science and the practice are not mutually exclusive. The practitioner 'on the job' needs to know about the evidence from carefully controlled studies. It will inform and contribute to decisions in practice. Equally he needs to be able to interpret those findings, taking into account the unique situation of the patient in front of him. This is where the skill or artistry of the professional is crucial. Equally importantly, he needs to be able to formulate the questions to which he needs answers, and these may not always be the questions which a randomized controlled trial will have addressed or be able to answer. Sometimes they will be questions about the context itself, for example about how and why the 'placebo effect' is so powerful or about how eye contact can affect the quality of a consultation. Often they will need to take into account qualitative as well as quantitative evidence, description as well as numbers.

Giving a context back to the research, considering the uniqueness of the situation in which a study has been done and the different contexts to which the results might be applicable are often the most challenging tasks, and we will consider them in detail in this book.

REFLECTION-IN-ACTION AND REFLECTION-ON-ACTION

Schon (Schon, 1983) distinguishes between reflection-in-action and reflection-on-action. The former occurs when a surprising or puzzling event makes you question what you are doing as you do it and this leads to a reshaping of responses during the action itself. There may be an internal dialogue (a 'reflective conversation') in which events and ideas mould each other during a clinical encounter. This is learning 'on the hoof' with experience directly altering behaviour patterns. Practitioners use critical appraisal skills during as well as after their clinical encounters. There is potential for this to expand in complexity as the new technology brings 'clinical decision support' to the consulting room.

Reflection-on-action has been described as a 'cognitive post mortem' although feelings as well as thoughts are relevant to such reflections. Here the practitioner looks back after the event to tease out the tacit assumptions and theories behind behaviour. Critical reading can help with the cognitive part of this by helping to consider available evidence. The process of reflection allows the evidence to be put into the context of the individual clinical encounter.

REFLECTION IS THE KEY

Such tasks are as important a part of critical reading for the practitioner as is the ability to appraise systematically the design, methods and analysis of a published study. We need something which will take the mystery out of critical reading and which will allow us to integrate the findings of research with the reality and uncertainty of primary care. We believe that reflection is the key to this process because it is a way of putting back the context, allowing a holistic approach and attempting to anchor research findings in reality (Fig. 2).

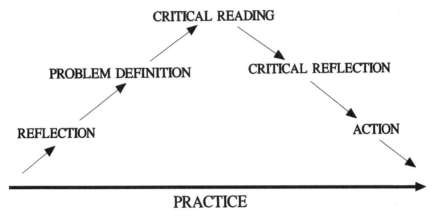

Figure 2. Reflection, critical reading and changing practice.

This emphasizes that a practitioner's experience is itself important and provides valid evidence from which questions arise and to which the findings of research might apply. Reflection is the artistic, subjective complement to the scientific, objective skills of critical reading. In other words, we need both the narrow rigorous approach of EBM and the reflective skills to put that evidence into context.

THE STRUCTURE OF THIS BOOK

We have divided the book into two sections. Critical appraisal and critical reflection are relevant to both. The first tackles the evaluation of an individual study. We review the main concepts we regard as helpful for critical appraisal and consider systematic ways in which the practitioner can critically reflect on a study. The second part focuses on how to select and use the literature on a topic where several papers may be relevant. Reflection here is used in a broader sense than in part one, for here the experience and knowledge of the practitioner helps to fashion the form and substance of the questions asked as well as the interpretation of answers which the papers may provide.

In both sections, we attempt to relate the examples we use to the experiences of those working in primary care. Many readers will want to read short sections of the book at one time. We have tried to give opportunities for readers to reflect on how the material presented may or may not be relevant to their own practice, and have suggested ways in which readers may be able to take forward

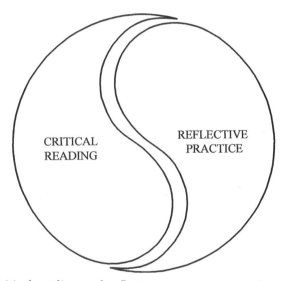

Figure 3. Critical reading and reflective practice as complementary processes.

their own learning and problem-solving agendas. The examples given and papers quoted will necessarily be out of date by the time this book is in print, so we must emphasize that they are only examples to show how the process of critical reading and reflective practice can be linked (Fig. 3).

SUMMARY

This book:

- is aimed at all practitioners working in primary care;
- provides a practical hands-on approach to the basics of critical reading;
- avoids jargon as much as possible (and explains it when it can't be avoided);
- offers a logical framework for relating research to practice;
- is based on the belief that reflection on your own practice will allow you to make the best use of evidence-based medicine and will stimulate your continuing professional development.

This book is *not*:

- designed as an introduction or guide to research;
- appropriate for those involved in systematic reviewing.

The skills of critical appraisal and critical reflection are necessary but not sufficient requirements for a practitioner who wishes to undertake research, and we hope that this book will stimulate the appetites of some of our readers to acquire the additional skills needed. Some have argued that primary care professionals are best

CONTINUING PROFESSIONAL DEVELOPMENT (CPD) IN PRACTICE

Based on report of CMO to the Secretary of State 1998

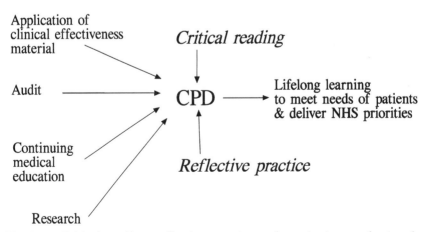

Figure 4. Critical reading, reflective practice and continuing professional development Calman (1998).

placed to judge the most relevant research questions to ask, but that most practitioners are quite rightly devoted to service provision, and research culture is not yet integrated into primary care. We hope that the development of reading and reflection will help the process of integration.

The majority of practitioners are more interested in service delivery than in either education or research. In writing this book, we aim to explore the basic skills for those who wish to reflect on their practice and improve their critical reading. We see critical reading and reflective practice as complementary processes which will help in continuing professional development (Fig. 4). We hope that reflection will allow practitioners to make the best use of the challenges of evidence-based medicine.

REFERENCES

Barnett, R. (1997) *Higher Education: A Critical Business*. Buckingham: Open University Press.
Calman, K. (1998) *A Review of Continuing Professional Development in General Practice*. London: Department of Health.
Schon, D.A. (1983) *The Reflective Practitioner*. USA: Basic Books.

Part I

Assessing an individual study: critical appraisal and critical reflection

1

What's the big idea?

This first chapter sets out some of the main ideas and themes in critical appraisal and critical reflection which we think are important. These ideas will pop up repeatedly in different contexts and examples throughout the book.

IDEA I: BROAD ISSUES NEED FOCUSED RESEARCH

Anton Chekhov, a doctor as well as a writer, tackled Life, Love, God, Death and Other Important Things by writing about highly select little corners of a society remote from ours in time and space. In stories often only a few pages long (Chekhov, 1984), he investigated broad issues, which are still relevant today, by describing particular incidents and particular people with precision and insight.

So it is, more modestly, with research. One general practitioner researcher, for example, wanted to compare two distinct and different styles of consultation (Thomas, 1987). When patients arrived to see him, they were allocated at random to receive one of the two approaches. The doctor then followed them up to investigate whether the style of consultation had influenced the speed with which the patients recovered from their symptoms. Such a study in one practice by one doctor can provide general insights into how attitudes and language in the consultation influence patient satisfaction and the outcome of illness. These insights may have implications far beyond the narrow context of the study itself, as Figure 1.1 illustrates.

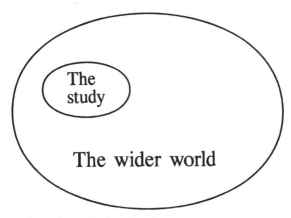

Figure 1.1 Small study, wide implications.

IDEA II: AN IMPORTANT DISTINCTION – WHAT HAS THE STUDY ITSELF DONE AND WHAT ARE ITS IMPLICATIONS?

The first task of researchers is to recognize a broad issue and from this to formulate a focused question. The next step is to design and carry out a study which will directly address this focused question. Finally, they must address how the results obtained from the specific study may be applied back to the broader problem from which they started.

The first task for the critical reader is to accept that the piece of research in front of them has its own narrow purpose which must be judged on its own terms: the *specific* methods and results of a *particular* study must be examined first. It is less helpful to say 'I wouldn't have done that study' or 'I would have answered the question by doing a different type of project'. The starting point is to take the authors' own particular study and consider the authors' aims and objectives. This is part of what we are calling critical appraisal.

Step I: critical appraisal

Look at the specific objective, methods and results of the study.

Once this first stage has been tackled, it is appropriate to move from the specific to the general. This is where the critical reader may reflect on the limitations of focusing on one specific question. There may well be other important questions which need to be answered. This does not represent a criticism of the specific study being considered, but may well limit its implications for the wider world. Drawing such implications involves the reader in making *judgements* about the importance of the specific work.

Step II: critical reflection

Judge and discuss the implications for the world outside the study.

Example: salt restriction to treat hypertension

Non-pharmacological treatment of hypertension is attractive when compared with drugs: less costly, fewer side-effects, avoids difficult decisions about medication for borderline hypertensives. One study (MacGregor 1989) involved a rigorous short-term regime of dietary salt restriction. The design was a randomized controlled trial of salt restriction versus no salt restriction in known hypertensives. The result showed that there was a greater fall in blood pressure after 4 weeks in the salt restriction group than in the control group who did not restrict their salt intake.

As **critical appraiser** (step I), you want to ask some questions about the trial design.
(Try to think of one and write it down before moving on).

In **reflecting critically** on the result (step II), you change to asking 'Is this worthwhile? Could I do it in my practice?'.
(Try to think of two practical problems of putting this result into everyday practice and note them down.)

Step I (appraisal) would consider whether differences in blood pressure between the trial groups at the end of the study resulted from the salt restriction rather than from flaws in the study design or from chance variation. If the critical reader is satisfied, then the researchers have done their job, i.e. investigated the specific question they set out to answer and done so in a way that stands up to technical scrutiny.

Step II (reflection) has a different purpose: to assess the relevance of the study to the 'real life' issues in treating hypertension. For example, could this degree of salt restriction be sustained for long periods? Would lesser degrees of salt restriction also carry some benefit? How costly would it be to achieve this dietary change? It might be costly in terms of cash, time, and people's need to have a well-balanced happy life as well as a healthy one.

Both step I and step II are about the **validity** of the study. In other words, how true is the result presented to us by this piece of research?

Truth is a difficult concept in science because it 'all depends' on the question being asked and on the methods used to answer it. Parallel to our distinction between the specific study question and the broader issues it addresses, is the separation of validity into 'internal' and 'external'.

● **Internal validity.** This is related to step I.

Jargon corner

Internal validity

Can I believe the result of the study? This involves critical appraisal skills to assess the design and methods used in the study.

Did the salt and hypertension study answer the question of whether severe salt restriction over 4 weeks in established hypertensives reduces blood pressure? For example, did the nurses who measured the blood pressures during the salt study know to which group each patient belonged or not? i.e. were the observations blinded? Such a flaw in the design might be big enough to make us question the result.

Internal validity is mostly about technical issues of research methods and analysis. If the nurses were aware of the group status of each patient, this knowledge might have influenced their measurements and thus reduced the internal validity of the study.

● **External validity** is related to step II.

Jargon corner

External validity

Assuming the result of a study is internally valid, how true is it for the wider world outside the study? This involves the skills of reflecting on the importance and practical relevance of the study.

The result from the salt study might be applicable to other established hypertensives who are willing to maintain a rigorous restriction of salt in their diet. However, such patients may only be a select minority of hypertensives and may require a large input of time and effort to make the regime work. Rigorous salt restriction might simply be unacceptable in the short or long term to the majority of hypertensive patients, and the study result may lack external validity for these patients. Lesser degrees of salt restriction might benefit blood pressure in a wider sample of hypertensive patients but this cannot be assumed directly from the results of this particular study.

External validity is as much about reasoning from the results and about constructive speculation as it is about technical judgements. It is closely linked to the step of drawing implications from studies. It is an important part of critical reflection because such speculation depends on knowledge and experience of everyday practice.

IDEA III: RESULTS ARE ALWAYS BIASED

The critical reader, bursting with armchair knowledge of research methods, can easily cut a destructive path through all papers in sight. The first try with the chainsaw is fun, and it is easy to create large gaping holes in published research. Every study is dirty to some extent: the perfect one does not exist. An expectation of black-and-white answers to every question can lead to the feeling that research is so flawed there is no point in doing it.

The crucial task is to judge the effect which any bias may have on results and on the implications of those results. How much can we deduce from the study *despite* the dirt?

Those who have actually tried to do research have an advantage here. They have insight into the many difficulties involved in trying to pin down aspects of the dirty world in order to obtain valid results. This should encourage a more positive, constructive approach to criticism. Put another way, critical readers should try to align themselves with the authors rather than confront or mock them.

Example: teenage smoking

A group of GPs in a country town want to estimate how common teenage smoking is in their practices. They send an anonymous questionnaire about current smoking habits to all 14-year-old schoolchildren in the area, after gaining ethical, school and parental approval. They report that 60% of the children replied.

Think about **internal validity**. If non-smokers are more likely to reply than smokers, the prevalence of smoking based on returned questionnaires in this group might underestimate its true occurrence. This is an example of possible **selection bias**.

Jargon corner

Selection bias

If the people actually studied are not 'typical' or representative of the group the researchers intended to study, this may bias the result.

Teenagers may not reveal their true smoking habits, even if they respond to the questionnaire. This is an example of **information bias**, referring to errors in the way study information is gathered. The way in which the smoking question was asked, for example, might have been confusing. There is a need to ensure that information gleaned from a questionnaire about smoking actually reflects what the teenagers' smoking habits actually are. There are various ways in which this might be done. For example a different method of information gathering, such as interviewing, might be used alongside the questionnaire in a sample of schoolchildren to test out the accuracy of what the questionnaire is providing, although this would not be anonymous.

Jargon corner

Information bias

A study result can be distorted from the 'truth' if there are errors or inaccuracies in the way information has been gathered.

The result of the survey is that 20% of responders report that they currently smoke. Despite the dirt, does this information reasonably reflect smoking habits among 14 year olds in this town? Even if the non-responders had different smoking habits, would that make much difference to the general result – namely, that a substantial number of 14 year olds in this town smoke?

Reflection stop

Suppose you decide that this information is reasonably reliable, is it useful to you – in a different place, a different practice?

Such reflection is partly about **external validity**: is this practice population sufficiently like yours to be able to generalize the result? It is not a criticism of the study itself if you decide it does not apply to your practice (although if the authors claim it is universal in its

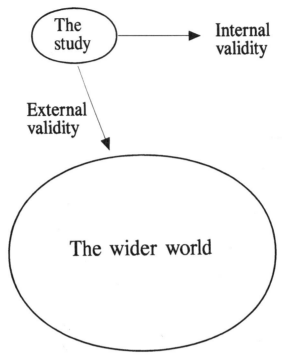

Figure 1.2 Internal and external validity.

truth, you may protest). It is also about considering the usefulness of the result and the wider application which it may have. The relationship between internal and external validity is illustrated in Figure 1.2.

IDEA IV: STATISTICS DO NOT EQUAL TRUTH

Statistics are the neurosis of the critical reader. Lacking the technical understanding, frightened by the jargon and the mathematics, overawed by the seeming monopoly on truth, the critical reader endows statistics with an undeserved power and magic.

The first and foremost job of statistics is to summarize the data from studies. The whole point of studying *groups* is to get a shorthand picture rather than rely on snapshots of every individual in the group. We should not lose sight of this basic and important function. This form of statistics is sometimes called *summary or descriptive* statistics.

The widespread fear of statistics has arisen because of *probability* statistics. These are sometimes called *inferential* statistics and refer to the role of mathematics in assessing the influence of chance. Such statistics cannot judge the truth of results or the relevance of results, but they can contribute to the evaluation of validity. In particular they give us an estimate of how chance might affect study results – how, for example, in a study of a small sample of all patients with hypertension, this might be the one occasion in one hundred when chance differences between the randomized groups have resulted in an apparent beneficial effect of salt restriction which might not be seen in 99 identical other experiments.

Chance, however, is only one element in judging the study – and not the most important. Remember that a statistically significant difference means simply and only that a result is unlikely to have arisen from chance alone. This will help in your assessment of the study, but tells you little about whether the result is clinically important or not.

Summary: the big ideas

I   Any one study has to focus on a small corner of the world; the critical reader does not dismiss it because of this but engages in a process of judging its relevance to the wider world.

II   The critical reader separates the broad aim and the precise objectives of the study and does not assess the paper for what it did not set out to do. The tasks are first to **appraise** the way the study has been done and second to **reflect** on its broader purpose, relevance and implications: in particular, how do the results apply to your own work, practice or patients?

III In reading critically, identify the really clean bits and reflect constructively on whether the grubbier aspects have useful things to say. Research is always flawed but it is also hard to do; we must get as much positive help from it as we can.

IV   Statistics are important but only contribute a part of the evidence. Logic and common sense are more important to the critical reader.

REFERENCES

Chekhov, A. (1984) The Early Stories 1883–88. Chosen and translated by Patrick Miles and Harvey Pitcher. London: Sphere Books Ltd.

MacGregor, G.A., Markandu, N.D., Sagnella, G.A., Singer, D.R.J., and Cappuccio, F.P. (1989) Double-blind study of three sodium intakes and long-term effects of sodium restriction in essential hypertension. *Lancet*, **(ii)**, 1244–7.

Thomas, K.B. (1987) General practice consultations: is there any point in being positive? *British Medical Journal*, **294**, 1200–2.

2

Summarizing a paper: an overview

In this chapter we review the component parts of a published research paper. Journals now help the process of identifying these components by publishing summaries or abstracts at the start of an article. The organization of this chapter follows the structure of such an abstract.

AIMS AND OBJECTIVES

The general aim

People do studies for all sorts of reasons. Those reasons may not be made explicit in a published paper, but this does not necessarily detract from the results. However, in the process of deciding on the importance of a set of results and their implications, you will need to consider why the study was necessary.

The topic of a paper may seem desirable to address in itself (such as the introduction of locally agreed guidelines for investigating infertility, or an audit of practice treatment for asthma). However, if the study is to evaluate or investigate these procedures, then the reasons for doing the study need to be clear. For example, a critical reader might include in their summary a precis of the introduction to one study of guidelines (Emslie, 1993) as follows: 'Guidelines are popular, but in the field of infertility they may lead to increased costs and demand on scarce resources with no clear benefit for patients. The authors therefore carried out a study. . .'.

Example: the risks of screening programmes in primary care

A study of the health effects of screening for cardiovascular risk took as its starting point the observation that GPs were being encouraged to undertake such screening (Stoate, 1989). The problem, as perceived by the author, was the lack of evidence that screening programmes were beneficial – and the possibility that they might have undesirable side-effects. For every patient identified with severe hypertension, for example, there might be many normal or borderline cases who suffer unnecessary anxiety as a result of the screening process itself. The author considered it was important to investigate the risks of screening to the health of fit people.

The specific study objectives

These arise from the general aim, but now the researcher is saying:

'Right, this is an important topic for research, what SPECIFIC question about the topic are we interested in asking, which will shed light on the general issue and which can actually be done in practice?'

This involves a narrowing of focus from the broad sweep of the general aim to the specific, clearly stated objective or objectives of the study. The objective of the cardiovascular screening study described above was as follows (Stoate, 1989):

'This study set out to determine whether cardiovascular screening offered to men and women aged 35 to 59 causes psychological distress in those who have normal findings at screening'

Note how the whole focus has narrowed down to set the boundaries of the project itself. This study is going to look at psychological distress – not absence from work, or alcohol consumption, or any other side-effect of a screening programme. You will have in the end to judge the relevance of this particular piece of work to the general issue under scrutiny, but you should only assess the methods and actual results (the **internal validity**) in the light of what the study has actually attempted to do, i.e. to investigate the effects of cardiovascular screening on *psychological wellbeing*.

Consider a second example: introducing guidelines for the management of infertility (Emslie, 1993). The aim of this study was put thus:

> 'We have carried out a randomised controlled trial of the introduction into general practice of agreed guidelines and recording sheets for use in the management of infertile couples, to determine the effect on subsequent fertility rates.'

This sets out an ambitious but clear objective – do guidelines result in a better final clinical outcome for patients? It would be no less valid to take a different outcome, for example do guidelines improve the standard of information which is given to the consultant in the referral letter? Such 'process' measures – so called because they take as a yardstick some improvement in the whole process of managing a clinical problem, rather than a measure of actual health (cure, palliation etc) – are perfectly reasonable targets for investigation, but they demand different studies with differently stated objectives.

Jargon corner

General aim: Why was the study done: what is its perceived general importance?

Specific objective: What is the specific question or questions being addressed by this particular study?

THE CONTEXT OF THE STUDY

This is concerned with two issues: where did the study take place (the **study setting**) and in what group of people was it carried out (the **study population**)?

The setting

Where was the study performed? This becomes important when you are thinking about generalizability of the results and their implications for primary care.

For example, in a study of obstetric care in Bradford (Bryce, 1990), the authors made some comparisons between perinatal outcomes in Bradford and outcomes observed in a study from Oxford. The social, cultural, economic and ethnic background to obstetric care in Bradford is likely to be very different to that in Oxford and may influence any differences observed in obstetric outcomes in the two settings. This will be relevant to the interpretation of the comparison.

The study population

The term 'population' is used in medical research papers in a technical sense – it refers to a group of people, as distinct from individuals.

Ask yourself:

1 To whom is it intended that the results should apply?
2 Whom did the researchers set out to study?
3 Who was actually studied?

Then ask how the researchers got from 1 to 3. This is important first in judging the internal validity of a study, and also when you move on to draw implications from results.

The way a group of people is selected for a study can give important initial clues about internal validity, especially when comparisons are being described. In a study comparing two groups of people, the researchers may have used different methods to select each group and this may have influenced the result. The critical reader must make an assessment of the extent to which such differences might have affected the internal validity of the study.

The randomized controlled trial tries to get round this problem completely by using random allocation to put study subjects into comparison groups. The underlying assumption in a randomized trial is that the two comparison groups have been selected in an identical fashion (i.e. by chance alone) and the only difference between them is that one group receives the study intervention and the other receives the placebo or comparison treatment.

Example: teenage smoking in two general practices

The important issue when summarizing a paper is to be clear about how the study groups were arrived at: this sets the scene for the critical appraisal. Take, for example, a hypothetical study comparing teenage smoking rates in two practices, one running a quit smoking policy and the other not. You note that in one practice the study population was a random sample of teenagers registered with the practice, of whom 50% responded to a postal smoking questionnaire. In the other practice the study population consisted of teenagers who attended the surgery during a 6-month period who were given a questionnaire by the receptionists and who completed it in the surgery. It was not clear in the second practice what proportion of all teenage attenders in that period were asked to complete the survey and how many of them actually completed and returned it.

Whatever analysis of the internal validity of this comparison you make later, the summary establishes that the study populations which are being compared were selected in different ways in the two practices. This is illustrated in Figure 2.1. In the second practice we do not know what proportion of those whom the researchers set out to study were actually studied. (**Selection bias** will be high on your agenda for appraisal here.)

Equally important is that the summary of how the study populations were selected will raise questions of **external validity**, i.e. the generalizability of the results.

Example: spinal manipulation for low back pain

A randomized controlled trial was carried out to compare chiropractic with 'usual' health service physiotherapy in the treatment of low back pain (Meade, 1990). The patients approached had all been referred to a chiropractic clinic by their general practitioners. They were asked if they would participate in a trial which might or might not mean that they would get chiropractic therapy, and as expected, some declined to take part in the study. Anyone suspected of a serious disease affecting the spine was excluded, and X-rays

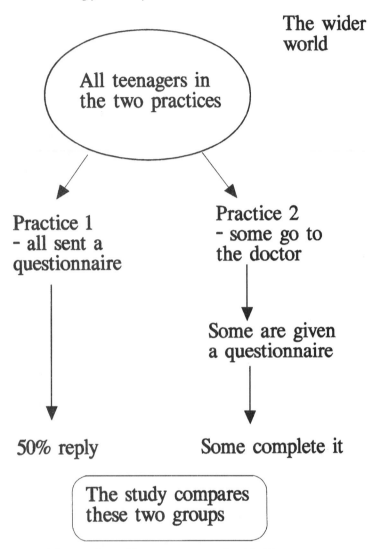

Figure 2.1 Selection bias: like not compared with like.

were performed on all those who agreed to take part in the study prior to their final inclusion. Those included were then allocated by a random method to (i) having the chiropractic therapy they had been referred for in the first place or (ii) going instead to a hospital physiotherapy department. The selection of the study population is summarized in Figure 2.2.

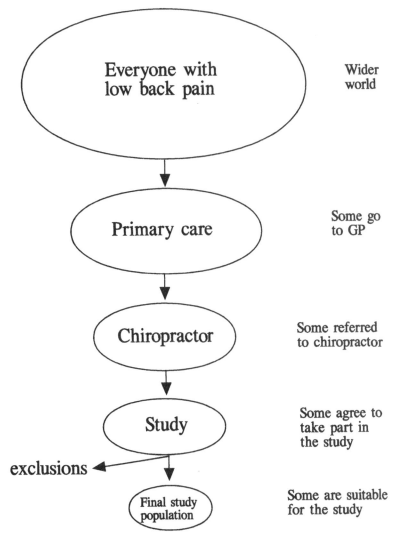

Figure 2.2 An example of selecting a trial population: the back pain trial.

The broad issue was whether one treatment worked better than the other. The narrower study question was whether chiropractic therapy worked better than hospital physiotherapy in a group of patients (i) who had agreed to chiropractic in the first place and (ii) who had agreed to take part in a trial and (iii) from whom those with radiographic abnormalities or serious problems had been weeded out.

Reflection stop

An important component of critical reflection is to think how the study population relates to your own patient groups. Before reading on, consider how the patients who were finally included in the spinal manipulation study might differ from the average low back pain sufferer in primary care.

In routine practice, patients may come in complaining of recent onset of low back pain, which in a relatively brief consultation you decide is unlikely to be due to any sinister underlying problem. You have essentially made a diagnosis of non-specific low back pain, for which you would be reasonably happy to recommend some form of physical therapy, be it treatment from a physiotherapist or manipulation from a chiropractor. If you use the results of this trial, and recommend chiropractic therapy, you are taking a step away from the context and rules that govern the trial itself. You have, for example, not carried out an X-ray and you are going to recommend manipulation rather than involve the patients in a detailed decision about whether they want to take part in a trial or not. This is perfectly legitimate and something that you may well have to do frequently. However, as a critical and reflective reader you must think through the implications of this. Implications such as the potential workload on a local service that might not initially be able to cope. Implications of the costs to the patient for paying for what might still be an exclusively private service. Implications for recommending manipulation in patients whom you are reluctant to X-ray on clinical grounds, even though the study demanded that everyone was X-rayed.

Most studies are carried out in a restricted sample of people, and can only address one aspect of the whole question being asked. The key step in summarizing a study is to be clear how that restricted sample was arrived at. This lays the basis for the reflective steps of critical reading, which will take the results of what has been done, by whom and to whom, and consider how these might apply beyond the confines of the study population itself.

Jargon corner

Setting: Where was the study done?

Study population: This refers to any group of people being studied.

a To what population do the authors intend the results to apply (the **target population**)?
b From what population did the researchers actually start (the **sampling frame**)?
c Who were the people finally studied (remember exclusions and refusals) (the **study population**)?

THE DESIGN

Spotting the design which has been used and putting a name to it is a crucial step in setting up a critical appraisal of the study itself. Now that summaries are often published at the start of a paper, the onus is on authors to decide what design they have used rather than on the reader to try to 'second guess' it. It helps considerably if you are familiar with the jargon of design. Some of the important terms are explained below.

'Intervention' or 'Observation'?

These terms might not be used but mentally you should bracket any study into one of these two groups. The basic question to ask is this: have the researchers introduced a treatment or procedure as part of the study? If so, this means you are dealing with an intervention study. This may have all sorts of implications for how you appraise results or conclusions, because an important feature of intervention studies is that the researchers have some control over how an intervention or treatment is introduced.

Example: vitamin supplements in pregnancy

The objective was to determine whether vitamins taken by women at the time of conception reduced the incidence of neural tube defects in the fetus (MRC Vitamin Study Research

Group, 1991). An intervention study allocated women at high risk of such affected pregnancies to receive active folic acid tablets or placebo tablets.

The alternative to intervening is to research and observe a slice of life or medical activity as it is – warts and all. Such **observational** studies may not be scientifically as pure as intervention studies but they are necessary, and many decisions in clinical medicine and public health utilize such studies. The fact that they take the situation as it is (rather than trying to manipulate it by introducing an intervention) does not mean such studies are simply anecdote dressed up for public appearance in a journal. Much effort has gone into developing methods of observational research to get round the problems which arise from not being able to carry out a classic 'scientific' experiment.

There are for example alternative strategies to the intervention experiment described above.

An observational study compared women who had been offered folic acid regularly when planning to become pregnant, with a group of women who had not taken the vitamin (Smithells, 1980). The outcomes of pregnancies in the two groups were ascertained and compared. The two groups were matched for other factors (such as age) which are known to affect the incidence of neural tube defects.

Jargon corner

Researchers can either observe things as they are or they can alter things on purpose to investigate the effect.

Hence a basic separation into **observational** and **intervention** studies.

The time frame: cross-sectional, retrospective, prospective?

These terms refer to the view of the researcher.

> A study set out to find out at one point in time how many children have neural tube defects in a group of practices. This is a cross-sectional view of the situation as it is at one moment or period in time.

Such surveys are important designs for assessing health needs, or the burden of disease which the health services are meeting or ought to meet, or the potential costs of looking after patients. It is a picture of the current state of affairs, a 'snap-shot'.

A prospective study means that the researcher sets a study up in such a way that he or she follows the study forward through time, collecting figures and data as events happen.

> A prospective observational study of folic acid and birth defects identified two groups of women, one taking the vitamin and the other not. The two groups were then followed forward over time to identify all women who had subsequent pregnancies affected by neural tube defects (Smithells, 1980).

The first advantage of prospective studies is that they get things in a logical sequence, in other words they try to put cause before effect. A second advantage is that it is possible to design forms for gathering data, and to decide on the information which needs to be collected, before the study starts. So, for example, an audit carried out prospectively with forms designed in advance may collect more complete information than a retrospective study which relies on going back through ordinary clinical case notes. The retrospective study in this situation has to use information which may be perfectly alright, but may not have been recorded systematically, and because it is retrospective there is often no way of knowing how much of it has been recorded.

Practicality often demands that a retrospective study is performed. The researcher must look back in time for the answer to the study question.

> Folic acid supplementation was studied retrospectively by identifying a group of women who had given birth to a child with a neural tube defect and then establishing whether they had taken the vitamin during pregnancy. This group were compared

with a control group of women who had experienced births uncomplicated by neural tube problems, from whom similar information was obtained. Such case-control studies are often retrospective in design.

Jargon corner

From the perspective of the researcher, a situation can be studied at one point in time, or looking back to what has already happened, or investigated into the future.

Hence a separation into **cross-sectional, retrospective** and **prospective studies**.

Another example which illustrates the relationship between cross-sectional, retrospective and prospective studies is shown in Figure 2.3. Each study addresses smoking in bronchitis, but each is asking a different question for which the chosen design is suitable. A cross-sectional survey aims to determine the prevalence of smoking and bronchitis in a population sample, and the proportion of people who both smoke and have bronchitis. A retrospective study selects the bronchitics identified in the survey, and looks back in their practice records to ask how many have consulted in recent years. A prospective study selects all the smokers from the survey and follows them forward in time to find out how many develop symptoms of bronchitis during the next 10 years.

Controlled or uncontrolled?

A crucial fact to establish is whether the study has involved a comparison between two or more groups. Most research does involve a comparison of some sort and the question must be put 'what is being compared with what?'.

In design terms this boils down to whether the study is controlled or not.

In the example of babies with neural tube defects, the first cross-sectional survey sought simply to establish the preva-

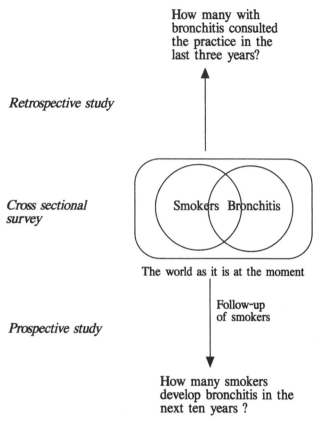

Figure 2.3 Three questions, three study designs.

lence of the disorder for purposes of needs assessment and care provision. Such a study does not require a control group – the figure for prevalence is complete in itself. If the researchers wished to report that the local prevalence was different to that in the general population, two groups would be compared (the study population with national figures as a control).

In the two observational studies of folic acid supplementation (prospective and retrospective), the theory that such vitamin supplements reduce the frequency of neural tube defects required that a control group was used for comparison (women who had not taken vitamins in the prospective study; women who had not had babies with neural tube defects in the retrospective study). These are both controlled studies, as is the intervention trial described in the first section.

Randomized or non-randomized?

This is an important question about controlled intervention studies. The key feature of a randomized intervention study is that the allocation of a particular treatment to any person who participates in the study is entirely random. The advantage is that differences between the groups can only have arisen as a result of two things: the intervention or chance. The role of chance here is an appropriate topic for statistical analysis.

The (folic acid) intervention study (pp. 33–4), in which vitamins were given to one group of women, would preferably have been carried out in this way. Non-randomized interventions are less appealing but may be needed for practical or ethical reasons.

> A hypothetical example of a non-randomized study would be a comparison of two towns. In this study all women living in one town and planning pregnancy were allocated to receive folic acid, while all women living in another town might be allocated to taking placebo. Here the comparison is between a policy pursued in one town and its outcome, and a policy being pursued in another town together with its outcome.
>
> The role of possible differences between the towns (other than the vitamin supplementation) which might affect the outcome would have to be taken into account. For example, it might be difficult to attribute a difference to the intervention if the sample of women given vitamins lived in rural Kent and the sample given placebo lived in inner-city Manchester. The socioeconomic mix will be different in these two places and this might influence the result because of contrasts in diet, smoking, antenatal care etc.

Summary box: design

The study design can be pinpointed by some keywords. Is it:

● observational or interventional?
● cross-sectional, retrospective or prospective?
● controlled or uncontrolled?
● randomized or non-randomized?

TEST YOURSELF: STUDY DESIGN

Question

Read the eight short summaries which follow and describe the design of each before reading the answers.

D1 **Intrapartum care**

A study set out to ascertain the relationship between intrapartum care provided by the general practitioner and subsequent birth complications (Bryce, 1990). Information was extracted from hospital records for the previous year. All deliveries were investigated in this way, and information about the GP Unit was compared with that from the consultant wards.

D2 **Steroid injections for tennis elbow**

A hospital team investigated the efficacy of steroid injections in the treatment of tennis elbow (Day, 1978). Alternate new patients with this problem, whom they saw in the outpatients' clinic, were injected with steroid; the other patients were injected with saline. They followed them up 1 month later to find out the cure rate.

D3 **Teenagers and contraception**

Teenagers' knowledge and use of contraception was investigated by a group general practice in an inner-city area. They designed and tested an anonymous questionnaire in a local secondary school. They then carried out a single mailing of the questionnaire to all children aged 13 to 16 years registered with their practice.

D4 **Parental psychiatric problems and childhood respiratory infections**

A study of the relationship between consultations about childhood respiratory illness and parental psychiatric problems was carried out in a group general practice. One hundred children who attended the surgery with upper respiratory infection were identified during the study period. Each time a doctor saw such a patient they selected the next name on the age–sex register, checking that the second child was from another family. The records of the parents of each pair of children selected were reviewed by a research worker to identify those taking psychotropic medication.

D5   **Styles of consultation**

A general practitioner attempted to find out what effect his style had on the outcome of a consultation (Thomas, 1987). When he saw patients with certain minor physical complaints, he would turn to a series of randomly ordered cards on his desk and turn over the top one. This informed him whether to adopt a directive or non-directive style of consulting behaviour.

D6   **Diabetic complications**

A group of general practitioners determined the rate of recorded complications in their diabetic patients by reviewing the records of all patients whose names had been placed on the practice diabetic register during the previous 5 years.

D7   **Infections and cervical smears**

A practice introduced a set of guidelines for the taking of swabs at the same time as cervical smears (Kelly, 1990). One year later they analysed the number of infections which had been identified from the swabs.

D8   **Shoulder pain**

A group of general practitioners from around the country decided to collaborate in finding out what happens to people who present with a new episode of shoulder pain (Croft, 1996). Each patient who attended with such a problem was entered on a register, and 6 months later a questionnaire was sent to them to ascertain whether they still had pain in their shoulders.

Suggested answers: study design

1   **Intrapartum care**

Retrospective:	Going back over records which had been collected before the study began.
Observational:	No intervention specifically undertaken for the study.
Controlled:	Results from the GP unit deliveries were compared with another group, namely deliveries in the consultant unit.

2 Steroid injections for tennis elbow

Prospective: Collecting patients and information after the study had started and as it progressed.

Controlled: Patients receiving active steroid injection were compared with a group receiving saline injections.

Non-randomized: Giving alternate patients the different injections may seem quite random, but in fact it is not a recognized 'safe' means of randomizing. Factors other than chance can influence such a process.

Intervention: A specific treatment was introduced as part of the study design.

3 Teenagers and contraception

Observational cross-sectional survey: A study conducted at one point in time, to assess some aspect of health in those surveyed, not involving a specific intervention as part of the study.

4 Parental psychiatric problems and childhood respiratory infections

Prospective: Patients were selected over time after the study had started, with the doctor aware that they were being included.

Observational: No intervention was included for purposes of the study itself.

Controlled: Records of parents of children who had not been to visit with upper respiratory infection were included to form a comparison group.

5 Styles of consultation

Prospective: The doctor involved consulting patients as part of the study.

Randomized: The cards naming the type of consultation style to be employed for a particular patient were ordered by a randomizing procedure, i.e. chance alone dictated which patients received which style.

Controlled: One style was compared with another style.

Intervention: The style was clearly a study intervention.

6   Diabetic complications

Retrospective: The doctors went back over records collected prior to the study.

Observational: This was a review of what had happened in the course of usual treatment and involved no study intervention.

Uncontrolled: This study was designed to produce a figure to describe the occurrence of complications in diabetics and no comparison was involved.

7   Infections and cervical smears

Prospective: Guidelines were introduced and the material to assess their effect collected subsequently as part of the study.

Intervention: The guidelines formed a specific intervention which was studied.

Uncontrolled: There was no comparison involved, for example with another practice.

8   Shoulder pain

Prospective: The study was set up prior to the identification of patients who could be followed up through time.

Observational: This was designed to describe what happened to shoulder pain sufferers with 'usual' treatment.

Uncontrolled: The group of shoulder patients was followed up and not compared with another group.

METHODS

Here the important thing is to identify the relevant methods, given the study objectives. Sorting out the design is the first step. Then the methods can be considered under three headings.

(i) For intervention studies: WHAT was the intervention and HOW was it carried out?

> For example, in the consultation study described in design question D5 above, how were the two styles defined? At what point in the consultation did the researcher introduce the designated style? Was the length of the consultation specified?

This is important both in judging the study itself (was the intervention rigorously specified or was it too vague to be assessed?) and in considering its implications (were the styles generalizable or was the whole thing too artificial to extrapolate?).

(ii) For all studies: WHAT was measured and HOW was it measured?

Here you will be interested first in baseline measurements (characteristics that were considered important enough at the start of the study to measure).

> For example, in design question D8, a prospective study of shoulder pain in primary care may want to investigate a number of potential influences on the outcome. So baseline measurement of age, duration of symptoms and initial treatment might be included.

Secondly there are outcome measurements (characteristics that are the main results of the study). Once again it is important to tease out exactly what was measured and how.

> For example, in design question D4, it would be important to know which psychotropics were included in the researcher's review and what details (time, duration, dose, number of

prescriptions issued) were recorded. Was the researcher extracting the information unaware of (or 'blinded' to) whether the records were from a parent of a child who had attended the practice with an upper respiratory tract infection or of a child selected as a control?

If there is a clear hierarchy of importance between multiple outcomes, they are often split into primary outcomes (related to the main objective of the study) and secondary outcomes (important but not essential to the main question).

Jargon corner

Baseline measures
Patient characteristics assessed at the start of the study, including general features such as age, sex and social class. They may be there for illustration, to allow comparability of study groups, or to study their influence on outcome.

Process measures
The way in which treatments or procedures are carried out in the study (e.g. number of visits, dose of drugs, types of swab taken). Their two main uses are to display the rigour of the research methods used and to allow an assessment of the generalizability of study methods.

Outcome measures
Those occurrences which the study has aimed to investigate (e.g. death, recovery, return to work, continuing disability). It is helpful if the authors have distinguished the most important ones (primary) from those which are interesting but not the main focus of the study (secondary).

(iii) Are the methods quantitative or qualitative?

In this book we are basing our main thoughts and arguments on traditional epidemiological and biostatistical approaches to medical research, the so-called quantitative methods. However, an increasing part of the research literature is concerned with qualitative methods of data collection and interpretation. Chapter 5 will briefly consider these.

Example: an assessment of health care needs among stroke patients in primary care

Patients with a history of stroke recorded on a practice morbidity register were sent a questionnaire about various aspects of their daily living, including any restricted activity, emotional problems, and dependency on carers. From this the proportion of stroke patients with problems which might benefit from interventions was identified. This helped the general practice in its planning of services for the future.

In addition a selected sample of individuals identified through the questionnaire as representing specific problems (lack of a carer, no contact with official services, complaints about proffered services) were visited and interviewed in depth by a trained qualitative researcher. Individual views, ideas, problems and suggestions were explored, together with those of other household members. This material aided interpretation of the quantitative figures obtained from the questionnaire. It also formed an investigation of some separate themes, such as the importance to some patients of being able to demonstrate a degree of independence from the health care system.

The two methods outlined in this example are not exclusive or incompatible, but their function is different, and in particular the methods of analysis and the process of generalization are different in each case. Quantitative methods are based on group characteristics, and rely on appropriate sampling and on enumerating those characteristics. Qualitative methods use the richness of individual patient's lives to understand general issues; they focus on patients' own narrative, on direct observation and on routine documentation as a basis for inferring what these issues mean to individual patients. They are no less rigorous than quantitative methods in the explicit descriptions of methods of subject selection and of analysis of material.

RESULTS

There are no specific rules about summarizing results, except that you need to identify the important and relevant ones. It is not unusual in a full-length research paper for results which are not germane to the central objective of the paper to appear. This may be for good reasons (for example to explore other factors which may have influenced the results) or for bad (padding out with irrelevant material). Your guide in describing the main results should be the *aim* and *objectives* of the paper which you have already identified.

For example, the tennis elbow study (design question D2), was not strictly randomized, and so a summary of baseline characteristics, such as age, sex and duration of symptoms, would be helpful to show that the two intervention groups were similar with respect to such features.

In the cervical swab example (design question D7), the number of smears showing carcinoma-*in-situ* in itself would not be an important result to include in the summary. However, the number of unsatisfactory or inflamed smears may very well be, if the purpose of the study was to determine the rate of infection in women presenting for smears and the effect that this has on the cytologist's ability to read the smear effectively.

Summary box

Methods: Include a clear statement of:

● the intervention if appropriate;
● baseline measurements.
● outcome measures: primary and secondary

Results: Summarize the main ones directly related to the purpose of the study (especially those involving the primary outcome measures). Beware of getting embroiled in subgroup analyses or details not relevant to the main question.

THE AUTHORS' CONCLUSIONS

It is important to differentiate between the authors' conclusions and your own. The authors' conclusions allow you to ask 'are they justified in their conclusions?'. To answer this you must critically assess the authors' reasoning. Your own *critical reflection* on the results will follow your appraisal of the whole paper, and this is dealt with in detail in Chapter 6. In summarizing a paper, it is sensible to focus first on the conclusions reached by the authors themselves and leave your own reflections until later.

Summary box

Conclusions: In a summary of a published paper these should be the authors' own conclusions.

Summary box: summarizing a paper

General aim: One sentence to say why the authors did the study: what was its importance as perceived by them.

Objective: What was the specific objective of this particular study?

Design: Try to pinpoint with a few well-chosen words!

Observation or intervention?
Cross sectional, retrospective or prospective?
Controlled or uncontrolled ?
Randomized or non-randomized ?

Context

Setting: Where was the study done?

Population: refers to any group of people being studied.
a To what population is the study to apply (the *target population*)?
b What was the starting population (the *sampling frame*)?
c Who were the people actually studied – remember exclusions – (the *study population*)?

Methods: Summarize briefly.

Intervention if appropriate
Baseline measurements
Outcome measures
Quantitative or qualitative

Results: Identify those directly related to the purpose of the study. Beware of subgroup analyses or details not relevant to the main question.

Authors' conclusions: Cover the main points made.

AND FINALLY: BACK TO THE CONTEXT

When reading a paper critically, it helps to bear in mind the general stages which precede publication of a piece of original research.

The stages of producing a research paper

1 A problem or issue is seen as important to primary care.
2 A specific question is formulated which might help tackle all or part of the general issue.
3 The planning and design of a study to address the specific question. A pilot study is often performed to check feasibility prior to the main study itself.
4 The study itself: interventions if relevant, data collection.
5 Analysis, presentation and publication of results related to the specific question.
6 In the discussion section the researchers will consider the flaws and the strengths of the study, and how they feel the specific question has been answered. Then, using the results from the

study, they may consider the extent to which the work has contributed to resolving the general problem or issue which initiated the project.

The stages of critical reading

The process of critical reading should follow the same route – from the general importance and significance of the subject being tackled, to appraising the particular piece of research displayed in front of you, and finally, using reflective skills, to the general context again to consider the implications of the results for the wider world of primary care.

When attempting a summary, the overall view of a paper in its context usually becomes apparent quickly. This is a very important aspect of critical reading which may sometimes be forgotten when

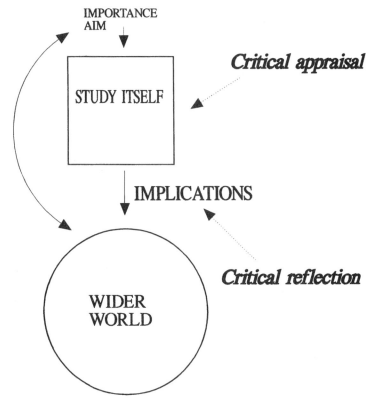

Figure 2.4 A study in its context.

it comes to the detailed critical appraisal of methods and results. The latter is all about 'Do I believe the results?', but the former is all part of developing skills of critical reflection to answer the question 'If the results are true, could they apply to my work, and how?'. This is summarized in Figure 2.4 which appeared in the introduction.

TEST YOURSELF: SUMMARIZING A PAPER
Question

Read the paper below (Stoate, 1989), and give yourself 20 minutes to write a summary along the lines described above. The abstract of the paper has intentionally been removed.

Can health screening damage your health?

Introduction
Adult screening for coronary risk factors in general practice is widely advocated on the grounds that it can save lives or at least reduce morbidity. Furthermore, it is believed that making people aware of risk factors will enable them to exert greater control over their own health. Advocates of screening tend to assume that there are only two possible outcomes of screening: benefit or no effect. A third possibility, harm, is frequently ignored. It can be argued that the debate about who to screen and for what conditions should be widened to take more account of its effect on a person's mental state and subsequent behaviour.

In order for screening to be of benefit it must be capable of detecting disease or potential disease not only before its usual clinical presentation but also before the point at which intervention becomes ineffective, sometimes called the 'critical point'. Unfortunately, relatively few medical conditions satisfy these criteria, and this may be one reason why many studies of adult health screening have had disappointing results. The Kaiser Permanente study failed to prove the case for multi-phase screening as opposed to conventional care. The authors of the south east London screening study found no good evidence of the usefulness of screening in middle-aged adults. Their conclusions were unequivocal: 'We believe that the use of general practice based multiphase screening on the middle-aged can no longer be advocated on scientific, ethical or economic grounds as a desirable public health measure'. The World Health Organization's European heart study showed no clear effect of screening on coronary heart disease end-points. Even the multiple risk factor intervention trial which looked at high-risk men aged between 25 and 57 years found no difference between 'special intervention care' and the usual community care over a 7-year period.

These trials all looked at hard end-points such as death or non-fatal myocardial infarction. None looked at the effect of screening programmes on the psychological state and behaviour of the participants. It has been shown by Haynes and colleagues that the labelling of previously undiagnosed hypertensives, detected by screening in the work place, results in increased absenteeism from work. It is therefore known that detecting abnormalities may have significant costs to the patient. What has not been studied is whether there are similar costs to people who do not have risk factors for disease.

This longitudinal controlled study in general practice looked at the effect of a by-invitation screening clinic on the psychological wellbeing of people found to have no detected abnormality, and thus labelled 'normal'. It was hypothesized that screening may make people more aware of illness thus increasing their psychological distress.

Method
The study was carried out in a new purpose-built six-handed practice in Bexleyheath, Kent. The practice employs a full-time preventive health worker who runs a by-invitation coronary risk screening clinic for men and women aged between 35 and 65 years. All patients in year of birth cohorts from the age–sex register were invited to make an appointment for a free health check.

The indicator of subjective psychological wellbeing used in this study was the 30-item version of Goldberg's general health questionnaire, a self-administered instrument which measures recent psychological distress, largely ignoring stable personality traits. It is ideal for general practice use, is simple to score, and has been shown to be sensitive to change over time. Subjects are usually considered to be minor psychiatric cases if they score above the cut-off score of 5. Although the instrument is designed to measure psychological distress, it has been shown to correlate with perceived health status.

Housing tenure was used as an indicator of social class. People were classified as living in owner-occupied, council rented or private rented accommodation. This information is obtained with a single question and is particularly useful in postal questionnaires. Previous studies have compared it favourably with the Registrar General's classification, and with socioeconomic group.

Between September 1987 and April 1988 attenders at the screening clinic were handed a general health questionnaire on arrival and asked to complete it before screening. Patients were then screened by the nurse who took a history of smoking, drinking, diet and family history of ischaemic heart disease. Blood pressure, height and weight were measured and urinalysis was performed. Blood was taken for lipids or liver function tests if appropriate. Any risk factors detected were discussed and advice and leaflets given if necessary. To look at the effect of screening on 'healthy' adults, patients found to have any of the following were excluded from the study: previously undetected blood pressure above 160/95 mmHg, newly detected glycosuria, fasting total cholesterol above 6.5 mM, or any other previously undetected abnormality which in the nurse's opinion required referral to the patient's doctor for further action.

Controls were randomly selected from the age–sex register using uninvited years of birth as close as possible to the study group, thus matching fairly closely for age. This group was sent a general health questionnaire by post with a letter asking for their help in a health survey. Reminders were sent after 10 days.

Subjects and controls were contacted in monthly batches of similar size in order to eliminate any seasonal effect on general health questionnaire score. This was achieved by selecting a larger control than subject group. It was reasoned that age–sex registers have a margin of error (10.5% in this case) and that response rates would be inevitably lower for a control group who gain no personal benefit from replying.

Subjects and controls both received a second general health questionnaire by post 3 months after the first, again with an explanatory covering letter. Reminders were sent to non-responders 10 days later.

Results

During the study period 234 people attended the screening clinic: 15 people (6.4%) were found to have previously undetected abnormalities and were therefore excluded from the study; two patients were in the process of moving house and two refused to take part: 215 patients were therefore enrolled. A total of 255 control patients were selected: three had been previously screened and 27 were unknown at their registered address: 225 controls were therefore included in the study. These were thus matched for age not sex. Interestingly, however, the groups had very similar sex ratios, indicating that there was no sex bias in attending for screening.

Response rates for the two questionnaires are shown in Table 2.1. The response rate of the control group to both questionnaires was lower than the study group. There was a

Table 2.1 Response rates for the two questionnaires

	Number (%) of patients		
	Enrolled	*Completed first questionnaire*	*Completed first and second questionnaire*
Study group	215	215 (100.0)	189 (87.9)
Controls	225	185 (82.2)	155 (68.6)

Table 2.2 Housing tenure of respondents

	Number (%) of respondents		
	Owner occupied	*Council rented*	*Private rented*
Study group ($n = 189$)	172 (91.0)	12 (6.3)	5 (2.6)
Control group ($n = 155$)	138 (99.0)	10 (6.4)	7 (4.5)

Owner occupied versus rented (private – council) $\chi^2 = 0.33$, df = 1, not significant

Table 2.3 Study and control group respondents with general
health questionnaire (GHQ) scores of 5 or more

	Percentage of respondents scoring >5 (95% confidence intervals)		
	First GHQ	*Second GHQ*	*χ^2 test with Yates' correction*
Study group (n = 189)	21.7 (15.2–26.8)	35.4 (28.2–41.8)	$\chi^2 = 8.10$ df = 1, $P < 0.01$
Control group (n = 155)	34.1 (26.6–41.4)	25.8 (18.0–32.0)	$\chi^2 = 2.21,$ df = 1, NS

close similarity in housing tenure between the study and control
groups (Table 2.2). The sex ratios of the two groups were also
similar with women comprising 56.6% of the study and 57.4%
of control groups ($\chi^2 = 0.049$, not significant).

When the general health questionnaire scores were compared for the two groups, there were two important results.
First, significantly fewer of those attending for screening had
psychological distress on the first questionnaire than the
control group (χ^2 with Yates' correction = 6.09, df = 1, $P<0.05$).
Second, significantly more of the screened group had a high
general health questionnaire score 3 months after screening
than before (Table 2.3). The control group showed a non-
significant fall in general health questionnaire scoring during
the 3-month period.

Discussion

The study demonstrated a significant increase in psychological
distress in healthy adults who have been screened for coronary
heart disease risk factors. An association, however, does not
prove causation – the effect may be due to selection or artefact
– and it is important to address some of the weaknesses of the
study design.

It is unfortunate that a smaller proportion of the control
patients completed both questionnaires, despite a postal
reminder, but it was felt to be important to avoid personal

contact by telephone in case this influenced the scores. The fact that fewer of those attending for screening had high initial general health questionnaire scores than the control group needs to be considered. It might be argued that anxious people or those with real or imagined health problems will be more likely to accept an invitation for screening. If so, we could expect a higher proportion of patients with high initial general health questionnaire scores, rather than the reverse. Attenders for screening are self-selected and certainly likely to be different from a random group of patients with similar socio-economic variables. The reasons why psychologically healthier people attend for screening is interesting and further work is planned to study this.

The decrease in scores for the control groups between the first and second questionnaires is the usual result seen with repeat administration of the general health questionnaire. What was totally unexpected was that significantly more of the study group had scores indicating psychological distress after screening than before. A study design can only eliminate known dependent variables and the higher general health questionnaire scores in the subject group may be a reflection of unknown variables. It is unlikely, however, that this could entirely explain significant differences between two fairly well matched groups. The possibility of a direct causal relationship between screening and increased stress cannot be ignored.

It is interesting to speculate about the nature of this relationship. The impression given by some patients was that receiving a letter warning them of risk factors for coronary disease and premature death made them feel that they had been negligent. This type of systematic screening may have made some people more aware of their mortality and more hypochondriacal, leading to greater psychological distress. If patients become more dependent on health services to deal with their life problems this has serious implications, not only for patients themselves but for the health services. General practitioners are being encouraged to screen more but Kleinman warned that as 90% of episodes of illness are dealt with without resorting to the doctor, a shift of only 10% in the proportion presenting to general practitioners would double our workload.

More work is needed in this area. Given that we have as yet no conclusive proof that screening alters the natural history of disease in a significant proportion of those screened, we must be cautious in our appraisal of measures which appear to reduce risk factors by detection and intervention. As Rose and Barker put it, 'The outcome of screening must be judged in terms of its effect on mortality and illness and not in terms of its restoration of biochemical or other test results to normal'. We must also address the possibility, previously largely ignored, that for some people at least, screening can do more harm than good.

Suggested answer: summarizing a paper

General aim

Screening for coronary risk factors is being advocated, but the evidence that it is beneficial is unclear and we do not know whether screening may actually be harmful to healthy people.

Specific objective of this particular study

To determine whether screening for coronary risk factors in general practice influences the subsequent psychological well-being of healthy adults.

The setting

A group general practice with a screening clinic.

The study population

a What was the target population?

Potentially all middle-aged people in Britain who might be called for coronary screening and given a clean bill of health.

b What was the sampling frame for this study?

Patients aged 35–65 years on the age–sex register of the study practice.

c Who were the people actually studied?

> One year of birth was selected at random from the sampling frame, and all names were sent an invitation to attend for coronary risk factor screening. The intervention group consisted of those who attended and were found to have no abnormalities on screening. The comparison group consisted of people in a second randomly selected birth-year who did not receive a screening invitation but who were sent and responded to a postal questionnaire.

Design

The study was a prospective randomized controlled intervention study.

Methods

The **intervention** was a coronary risk factor screening carried out by the full-time practice preventive health nurse at a special session, which included general advice on lifestyle from the nurse following a normal screening.

The **baseline measure** of psychological status was self-completion of the General Health Questionnaire (GHQ), which provides a score of probable psychological distress. It was given to the intervention group on arrival at the clinic prior to screening. It was sent to the control group by post.

The **main outcome measure** was psychological status as measured by the GHQ, sent by post to both groups 3 months after the baseline measurement.

Results

Patients in the intervention group had lower mean baseline scores of psychological distress than the comparison group.

The intervention group had a mean score of psychological distress at follow-up that was higher than their baseline mean. The comparison group mean had fallen on the second occasion compared with their own baseline.

Author's conclusions

The author states that the results need to be replicated, but, if true, then screening may have important deleterious effects on the psychological well-being of the large numbers of healthy adults who attend for coronary risk factor screening and are told they have no major risk factors. This has potential implications for clinical workload in general practice.

REFERENCES

Bryce, F.C., Clayton, J.K., Rand, R.J., Beck, I., Farquharson, D.I.M., and Jones, S.E. (1990) General practitioner obstetrics in Bradford. *British Medical Journal*, **300**, 725–7.

Croft, P., Pope, D., and Silman, A. (1996) The clinical course of shoulder pain: a prospective cohort study in primary care. *British Medical Journal*, **313**, 601–2.

Day, B.H., Grovindasamy, N., and Patnaik, R. (1978) Corticosteroid injections in the treatment of tennis elbow. *Practitioner*, **220**, 459–62.

Emslie, C., Grimshaw, J., and Templeton, A. (1993) Do clinical guidelines improve general practice management and referral of infertile couples? *British Medical Journal*, **306**, 1728–31.

Kelly, B.A., and Black, A.S. (1990) The inflammatory cervical smear: a study in general practice. *British Journal of General Practice*, **40**, 238–40.

Meade, T.W., Dyer, S., Browne, W., Townsend, J., and Frank, A.O. (1990) Low back pain of mechanical origin: randomised comparison of chiropractic and hospital outpatient treatment. *British Medical Journal*, **300**, 1431–7.

MRC Vitamin Study Research Group. (1991) Prevention of neural tube defects: results of the Medical Research Council Vitamin Study. *Lancet*, **338**, 131–7.

Smithells, R.W., Sheppard, S., Schorah, C.J., Seller, M.J., Nevin, N.C., Harris, R., Read, A.P., and Fielding, D.W. (1980) Possible prevention of neural-tube defects by periconceptional vitamin supplementation. *Lancet*, **1**, 339–40.

Stoate, H.G. (1989) Can health screening damage your health? *Journal of the Royal College of General Practitioners*, **39**, 193–5.

Thomas, K.B. (1987) General practice consultations: is there any point in being positive? *British Medical Journal*, **294**, 1200–2.

3

Can I rely on the methods? Issues of measurement

Choice of what and how to measure in a study is dictated firstly by the purpose of the study.

- A study of the effect of different non-steroidal anti-inflammatory drugs on the progression of osteoarthritis of the hip used radiological measurement to define osteoarthritis.
- A study of the effects of physiotherapy in patients with knee osteoarthritis used pain severity and restriction in activities of daily living to define the clinical problem.
- A study of the influence of occupation on lower limb osteo-arthritis used admissions to hospital for joint replacement to define severe disease.

It is wrong to suppose that there is an absolute correct way to define osteoarthritis for research purposes. This is obviously not so – the choice of definition depends on the specific research question being addressed.

Choice of measurement methods is also dictated by the design of the study.

- A practice-based physiotherapist's trial of bandage-taping the knee to reduce pain in patients with knee osteoarthritis used a visual analogue scale of pain severity from which a 'score' of pain can be derived. This information was gathered at baseline and 6 weeks after the intervention.

● A health visitor's study of the services provided for patients with knee osteoarthritis was based on a series of open-ended in-depth tape-recorded interviews with a small group of patients, selected from the practice morbidity register.

There are different ways to measure osteoarthritis or to define pain or to collect information about services: none are 'right' or 'wrong', and all are chosen in relation to what the study is about.

There is a large literature on the technical aspects of measurement in research. It is not our intention here to review these but to highlight certain issues which are important when assessing the methods used in any study. It is useful to recall one of the 'big ideas' in critical reading: the distinction between the study itself and the wider world, between **internal** and **external** validity.

ARE THE MEASURES RELEVANT TO THE STUDY OBJECTIVE?

Do all the measurements included in the methods section of a paper appear in the results section?

> ### Example: antibiotics and streptococcal pharyngitis
>
> In a trial of different antibiotic regimes for streptococcal pharyngitis in primary care, the introduction and methods sections of the paper emphasized that compliance with therapy and acceptability of the regimes were important outcomes (Shvartzman, 1993). No results appeared for either.

Remember that **outcomes** can be classed as primary (i.e. related to the main purpose of the paper) or secondary (i.e. important outcomes, but not the central focus of the paper). In general the study itself should be judged first on the basis of the primary outcome.

> In the pharyngitis trial (Shvartzman, 1993), bacteriological evidence of streptococci on culture of throat swabs was the primary outcome. Whatever you, the reader, feel about the importance or relevance of this outcome as a reason for treating sore throats in primary care, you must first appraise and judge the paper on its own terms, i.e. as an assessment of

the effect of different treatments on streptococcal cultures from throat swabs.

As the critical reader moves on to consider the implications or external validity of a study, it is often the secondary outcomes which become the main focus of interest.

In the pharyngitis trial, knowledge of the practical outcomes (treatment acceptability and compliance) is essential to a broader interpretation of the study, regardless of the main findings. These results were not given.

HOW WERE THE MEASUREMENTS CHOSEN OR DERIVED?

For all measurements which appear in the results section, is there a clear account given in the methods section of how they were derived?

This is a common problem. It does not require a technical knowledge of the methods involved to make a common sense judgement about it.

In the pharyngitis study, school or work absence was included in the results section, but no details were provided about how this information was obtained.

In a study of referral letters to orthopaedic departments and the corresponding replies (Jacobs, 1990), the contents of the letters were summarized in the results section by a 'weighted score' for each item in the letter. The rationale for the weighting was nowhere to be found in the methods. 'Scores' and 'weights' can be simple or they can be derived in a complex way. In either case there should be a clear and explicit basis provided for using them.

WERE THE SAME MEASUREMENTS USED FOR ALL GROUPS STUDIED?

In all studies which involve a comparison between two or more groups, has the information been derived or measured in the same way in all the groups?

Example: diet and breast cancer

Consider a hypothetical study of possible dietary causes of cancer. Breast cancer patients in hospital were interviewed about their dietary habits during the previous 5 years. A control group were also asked about diet: they were selected from women in the same hospital, admitted with benign gynaecological problems.

The measuring instrument was a semi-structured dietary questionnaire administered by a trained interviewer. It relied on the recall of the person being interviewed.

The **instrument** itself (i.e. the interview schedule) may not have provided an accurate reflection of the women's true diets during the previous 5 years. It can be argued that this weakness would apply equally to both study groups (cases and controls), but if recall is very poor, the comparison will be weak.

The information provided by the **study subjects** may have been influenced by their status: breast cancer patients may recall diet in ways which differ from the recall of women with non-malignant gynaecological problems because, for example, they are searching for a reason for their disease, or may have changed their diet in response to their diagnosis. This is an example of **information bias**.

The way in which information was collected by the **study observers** may have been influenced by the status of the subjects. It would be difficult to ensure that interviewers were unaware of any patient's diagnosis, although they might have been unaware of specific hypotheses about diet and breast cancer. The way in which information was obtained may thus have been different for cases and controls, another example of information bias.

These are all issues of internal validity. If groups are being compared with respect to some characteristic, it is a central issue of research methodology that the measurements are carried out in a standard way in all the groups. Otherwise information bias may creep in.

Jargon corner

Information bias

The measuring instrument can get it wrong (**instrument bias**), e.g. a faulty sphygmomanometer used in a community survey of blood pressure.

The people doing the measuring can get it wrong (**observer bias**), e.g. in the community survey of blood pressure, one researcher records the diastolic blood pressure when the sound starts to fade, the second researcher records it when the sound disappears.

The people being measured can get it wrong (**subject bias**), for example in the blood pressure survey, subjects are asked if they have had their blood pressure measured during the previous five years – those who are fit have poorer recall than those who have chronic illness.

A randomized trial of treatments for major depression in primary care compared brief psychological intervention with antidepressant therapy and with placebo drugs (Mynors-Wallace, 1995). Among the outcomes were 'observer and self-reported measures of severity of depression and psychological symptoms at 6 and 12 weeks'. Assessments were made by 'one of two experienced research interviewers who were blind to the type of treatment given'.

This paragraph gives all the relevant information. Because the interventions were so different (brief counselling versus tablets) it is important to be clear how the outcomes were measured. More than one method of measurement was used (self-report and observed). So, for example, an effect of counselling on patients' own reporting of their symptoms may not be found in the observer assessments. By contrast, awareness of treatment might influence the observers' assessments and so they remained 'blinded' to this.

Such practical steps reassure the reader that efforts have been made to ensure comparability of information gathering between treatment groups.

In the pharyngitis study (Shvartzman, 1993), nurses phoned the patients each day to enquire about compliance. No details were given about how the questions were asked, nor whether the nurse and the patient were aware (at the time of the call) of the treatment being received.

There are two levels of concern about outcome measurement in this example. First, the simple lack of detail. If you are not given the information, you cannot judge the quality of the outcome measurement. A simple rule here is to ask: 'Is the detail sufficient that I could repeat the study myself?'.

Second, telephone enquiry may be a flawed method of measuring patient compliance with treatment. However, before rushing to judgement, always ask the question, 'Would this have made any difference to the study result?'.

If both nurses and patients were unaware of the treatment group when the phone calls were made, an inaccurate method of assessing compliance may not matter, because the error would affect both groups equally.

If the compliance information is very weak, however, you might reason that the study will not contribute any meaningful realistic information about likely differences in compliance between the two treatments.

One point about the study was to compare a once-daily regime with a four-tablet-a-day regime. It seems unlikely that the interviewer could maintain a determined ignorance of the regime that any particular patient was on.

WHAT DOES THE MEASUREMENT ACTUALLY MEAN?

Does the measurement reflect what it is supposed to reflect? This is the most important question of all, and relates to the world outside the study (external validity).

There are two separate issues:

(i) Is the measurement technically a good measure of what it is supposed to measure or might it be biased?

The technical issue is one of 'gold standards'. This was raised in the breast cancer and diet example above: how true a reflection of actual diet in the past 5 years was the memory-based interview?

In a study of the influence of poster material displayed in practice waiting rooms (Ward, 1994), the length of time for which a patient had had to sit and wait before being seen was an important variable (the longer the time, it was hypothesized, the more likely the full contents of the posters would be absorbed). The waiting time was measured by asking the patient how long they had had to sit in the waiting room.

This might be a perfectly legitimate way to measure waiting time, but a more objective assessment would be needed to verify this. For example, recording of actual times by practice staff in a sample of the patients would help to judge the usefulness of recalled waiting times.

The choice of 'gold standard' depends on the study and its purpose. Phrases such as 'previously validated questionnaire' imply that some testing against a gold standard has been done. However it should be remembered that much of what we deal with in primary care is not 'measurable' in a traditional quantitative sense nor are there 'gold standards' in a strict sense. Do not demand of a study more than it sets out to deliver.

The National Morbidity Studies in primary care are carried out every 10 years in a volunteer sample of general practices in Britain (Royal College of General Practitioners, 1995). Diagnoses are recorded for every contact made with patients during the course of a year. They provide a major source of descriptive data on common symptoms and diseases in the community.

A criticism levelled at these studies is that a statistic based on, for example, the incidence of consultations for osteoarthritis in primary care is of little use because general practitioners often have no firm basis on which to diagnose osteoarthritis. The term might simply be a convenient label for pain in a joint. The purpose of a study might actually be to explore this very point: how does a general practitioner's diagnosis of osteoarthritis relate to radiographically defined disease? The diagnosis is thus tested against an outside standard, namely radiographs.

However this is not the only question of interest nor is radiology the only relevant yardstick for osteoarthritis. The incidence of consultations for what general practitioners diagnose as osteo-arthritis' may be a relevant measure for certain questions, for example the costs and benefits of using non-steroidal anti-inflam-matory drugs for joint pain which is clinically diagnosed as osteoarthritis.

(ii) Even if the measure is technically a good one, what does it mean in practice?

> In the paper on treatment of major depression in primary care (Mynors-Wallace, 1995), two of the outcome measurements used were the Hamilton rating scale for depression and the Beck depression inventory. These are instruments for assess-ing probable depression which have been validated against a psychiatrist's clinical interview and which produce a score. The scores in the study were found to be significantly different between the treatment groups, and the conclusion was that active treatment influences depression severity.

However, the authors were careful to look beyond the score. Did the changes observed in the scores reflect clinically important changes in the patients' condition? Change in a score was translated in clinical terms.

This example raises an important issue as the number of outcome measures multiplies and they become ever more sophisticated. For example, there is now a wide range of questionnaires to assess general health status. These have been used across a range of conditions and studies, which aids the process of comparing results. However, in drawing implications from studies which utilize such instruments, the critical reader must ask what these scores actually mean in practice in individual patients' lives. This is about critical reflection: extrapolating from an experiment to something which has a practical clinical interpretation or which means something to the individual patient.

> From the pharyngitis example, how relevant is eradication of streptococcus from patients' throats as the main purpose of the primary care of patients with sore throat?

In the orthopaedic letters study (Jacobs, 1990), how do scores of the content of letters translate into practice – what practical suggestions for change would arise from a statistical difference in the scores?

Jargon corner

Systematic error: Any regular distortion of a measurement away from what it is intended to measure.

Random error: Chance fluctuation in measurements which might influence the result of the study.

Sources of error: Instrument, observer and subject.

Repeatability: How consistent are measurements on different occasions:

- by the same observer (within or intraobserver);
- by different observers (between or interobserver).

There may be systematic or random elements to observer repeatability. These are often summarized by the kappa statistic.

Validity: How true is the measurement with respect to what it is trying to measure? Internal validity relates to the study itself and external validity to the outside world. If there is systematic error in repeatability then this will affect validity. However, a measurement can be perfectly repeatable and yet be invalid because it is not measuring what it is supposed to measure.

The difference and relationship between systematic and random error, repeatability and validity, is best summed up visually. Figure 3.1 is one found in many methods textbooks. The 'bullseye' is the 'true measurement'.

High validity means that overall the measurements approximate to the truth. Poor repeatability alone may reduce validity if random error distorts the average of the measurement. Low validity means the measurements do not reflect the truth: good repeatability does not necessarily correct this.

Repeatability

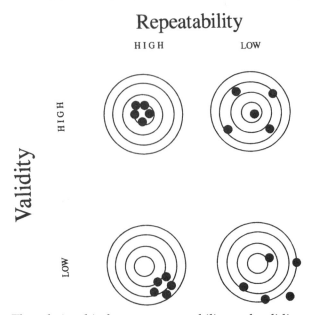

Figure 3.1 The relationship between repeatability and validity.

Summary

The two-step approach to a critical view of measurement:

1 How well has it been done? (**internal validity**)
2 How useful and relevant are the measurements? (**external validity**)

TEST YOURSELF: MEASUREMENT

The rate of consultation for asthma in the Royal College of General Practitioners' National Morbidity Survey increased from 9 per 1000 patients in 1971 to 16 per 1000 patients in 1981, and the rate of consultation for hay fever rose during the same period. This result was taken as evidence that allergen sensitivity or exposure had increased during that decade. The survey is carried out every 10 years and lasts for 1 year, involving doctors in almost 200 practices who record every patient contact during the study year.

Question

Comment on this result: can you think of alternative explanations of the result?

Suggested answer

This was a well-performed survey, based on a large number of recording practices. It has a reasonable conclusion, given hypotheses about changing allergen sensitivity in the modern world. This was a comparison across time: between a general practice population in 1971 and 1981. So was like being compared with like?

One possibility is that different practices took part in the two study years, and diagnostic behaviour was different in the two groups. More likely is that there was a general shift over time in general practitioners' habits of diagnostic labelling. Whatever the many and varied reasons – availability of better therapy, patient awareness, better diagnostic tests – it is likely that doctors' willingness and readiness to use the label 'asthma' altered during those years. A shift from vaguer notions of 'wheezy bronchitis' or 'chesty colds' might explain an apparent upturn in incidence of disease among consulters. Similar influences may have encouraged the use of hay fever as a diagnosis.

There are other possibilities: that it represents a rise in consultations by people who would not have consulted with the same symptoms in 1971 (patient awareness of diagnosis and treatment availability), or a real increase in asthma incidence in addition to changes in consulting or labelling patterns.

Note that we do not have to evoke the 'gold standard' argument, for example, that asthma can only be diagnosed after full investigation in hospital. The study was about 'asthma as it is diagnosed by general practitioners' and this is perfectly reasonable. However, since asthma defined in this way may have altered because general practitioners have altered their diagnostic behaviour, it may be a biased study of change in true incidence of asthma. There is possible information bias because what was measured in 1971 was different to what was being measured in 1981.

REFERENCES

Jacobs, L.G.H., and Pringle, M.A. (1990) Referral letters and replies from orthopaedic departments: opportunities missed. *British Medical Journal,* **301**, 470–3.

Mynors-Wallace, L.M., Grath, D.H., Lloyd-Thomas, A.R., and Tomlinson, D. (1995) Randomised controlled trial comparing problem solving treatment with amitryptiline and placebo for major depression in primary care. *British Medical Journal,* **310**, 441–5.

Royal College of General Practitioners and Office of National Statistics. (1995) *Morbidity studies in a general practice 1981–1982.* London: HMSO.

Shvartzman, P., Tabenkin, H., Rosentzwaig, A., and Dolginov, F. (1993) Treatment of streptococcal pharyngitis with amoxycillin once a day. *British Medical Journal,* **306**, 1170–2.

Ward, K., and Hawthorne, K. (1994) Do patients read health promotion posters in the waiting room? A study in one general practice. *British Journal of General Practice,* **44**, 583–5.

4

Can I believe the results?
Bias and confounding

WHAT IS BIAS?

Our attempts at medical research are efforts to represent or replicate what happens or might happen out there in the dirty, chaotic, unpredictable world of people falling ill.

The statistician in the mortality department is trying to count deaths in as accurate a way as possible; the practice nurse constructing a picture of his or her diabetic workload tries to identify the diabetics treated by the practice; the sociologist interested in carers' perspectives on the need for services for the disabled builds a narrative based on hours of interviews with a small group of carers; the practice manager tries to measure the effect on practice staff of altering the appointment system.

All will fail if they aim to produce a single absolute 'truth' about the question they have set out to answer. Their results will be approximate and will deviate from reality to a greater or lesser extent. Such results will not necessarily be less helpful for all that. Critics who will only believe or act upon studies which provide the absolute truth are not merely harsh judges – they are condemned to a life of total inertia. Worse still they are committed to whatever is happening at the moment in the real world – good or bad – because change on the basis of any research is impossible. The research will never come up to scratch.

So is the alternative to accept all research uncritically, on the basis that some evidence is better than no evidence, and some of the answers are likely to be true? The answer is no. The art of critical appraisal in medical research (by researcher and reviewer) is to ask:

- how might the study have deviated from the truth?
- how far might it have deviated?
- how has it avoided such deviation? and
- would any deviation have distorted the result?

This last question is the crucial one, and this is what **bias** is all about – not whether the result is a bit dirty and so may not be a perfect reflection of the truth, but whether it is likely to convey a systematically false picture of reality. As the late Professor Rose put it, dirt in research is not a problem if it is clean dirt (the truth is not distorted); it is a problem if it is dirty dirt (bias is present which has distorted the truth).

An example of bias and how to approach it

A nurse practitioner wishes to survey the lifestyle of adult patients in her practice to get a picture of their current smoking, exercise and dietary habits. She decides to mail a questionnaire to all adults on the age–sex register. This survey has a 70% response rate. Can she rely on the results of these responders as providing an accurate picture of what is happening in the whole practice?

A traditional answer was 'let's ask a statistician whether this is a good response rate'. However, there is a more thoughtful and productive approach, which does not demand such a black-and-white answer. Ideally the only 'true' reflection of the lifestyle of the population, as determined from a questionnaire, would come from a 100% response. This has not happened. There is no intrinsic problem with a 70% response so long as the 30% who have chosen not to respond (cannot read, bored with questionnaires, forgotten, too busy, intrusive) happen to have identical lifestyles to the responders. The picture obtained from the responders would then be true for the whole practice.

However this assumption is unlikely to be true. Research has shown that those who complete lifestyle questionnaires have different lifestyles to non-responders. Smokers may be rather less willing to tell the doctor about their habit than non-smokers are to reveal all about their abstinence. People who complete diet questionnaires are more likely to be those who have just virtuously wiped away the last fragments of muesli and brown bread from their lips than those who have finished off a bacon and fried egg sandwich. This is an example of **selection bias**. The bias is not the incomplete response itself, but the distorted picture which the completed questionnaires give of the lifestyles of the target population (i.e. the whole practice population). So do we reject the study? If we did, then no survey would be admissible on our terms unless there was a 100% response.

Investigating selection bias

Example: How different are non-responders?

(i) By maximizing the response, e.g. with reminders and repeat mailings in a postal survey

(ii) By gathering information by different means in a small sample of non-responders, e.g. by telephone or interview, and comparing with a similar sample of responders

(iii) By comparing other characteristics of responders and non-responders (e.g. age, social class) to determine how different they are.

It is important that critical appraisal is thoughtful and that a study is not crudely rejected because it only had a 50% response for example. The appraiser must ask some questions.

Judging the importance of bias

1 How large is it?
2 What effect might it have on the study result?

Bias comes in two varieties

There are many types of bias – one well-known publication identifies and names some 50 varieties (Sackett, 1979). Fortunately this encyclopaedic approach is not necessary to a critical reading of papers. Bias in fact boils down to two broad types – selection bias and information bias (Kopec, 1990).

The example of survey non-response above is one type of selection bias. Remember, non-response itself does not have to cause a bias. Only if it distorts the result from the 'truth', is it a potential source of bias.

SELECTION AND DROPOUT BIAS

Selection bias can apply to the initial selection of who was included in the study. In the survey example above, consider what would happen if questionnaires had not been mailed to all the practice, but instead were handed out to all patients who attended the surgery during a 4-week period. This method of obtaining information from patients in a practice is superficially attractive because of its high response rates. A questionnaire completed there and then in the waiting room can overcome some of the practical or psychological barriers to participation in postal surveys.

Again the relevant 'bias' question is whether the non-participants were different from those who had visited the surgery and completed questionnaires? Specifically, will the lifestyle of consulters be the same as the lifestyle of the whole practice population? This is unlikely, since consulters are more likely to be ill, and lifestyle and illness and consulting behaviour are all intertwined.

Does this matter? Such a question needs to take into account the objective of the study. If the researchers wished to identify a group of patients with poor physical activity levels to take part in an intervention study of exercise prescription, this form of selection might be fine (internally valid), although it may affect the generalizability (external validity of the results) and the implications that can be drawn.

Selection bias also applies to randomized trials and follow-up studies. Selection bias which affects internal validity in trials is usually about selective loss to the study, i.e. dropout and the reasons for it. It is a parallel situation to non-response. There may be so many dropouts that nothing can be concluded from a study, but usually the important question is whether those who dropout are different to those who stay in with respect to the outcome of the study being measured.

TEST YOURSELF: SELECTION BIAS

Question

Read the following and comment on any possible sources of bias.

> Patients attending surgery during the period of 1 month are asked to complete a physical activity questionnaire. All those who are taking minimal exercise and are considered suitable by the GP are invited to participate in a randomized controlled trial of a short educational intervention designed to encourage brief regular exercise each week. Those who agree are allocated on a random basis to receive or not receive the intervention. Three months later the practice nurse follows up both groups at a special clinic: 90% of those who did NOT receive the intervention turn up, compared with 60% of those in the intervention group.

When you have committed yourself to paper, read on.

Suggested answer

Note first that selection into the study does not raise problems of study bias. A group of patients with poor physical activity levels attending the surgery and considered suitable by their GP and willing to participate were then allocated to two comparison groups. This selection might be difficult to generalize if, for example, most of the patients with low physical activity were considered unsuitable for the trial or did not wish to participate – but this is not an issue of bias within the study (internal validity). As always with selection and participation, there is also the practical issue of numbers – if too many are excluded or refuse to participate, then the study may not get off the ground.

Bias becomes relevant at follow-up. Dropout occurred but is it different in the two groups? Certainly there is a different dropout rate in the two groups, but this may not be a bias if the reasons for dropping out are similar in the two groups. The important question is whether dropout is related to both intervention (advice to take exercise) and outcome (compliance with the advice). Bias will occur in the intervention group if those who do not turn up after 3 months are those who have not been exercising. In the 'treatment' group the successful ones return; whereas in the control group no such selectivity operates in the absence of an intervention. A spurious

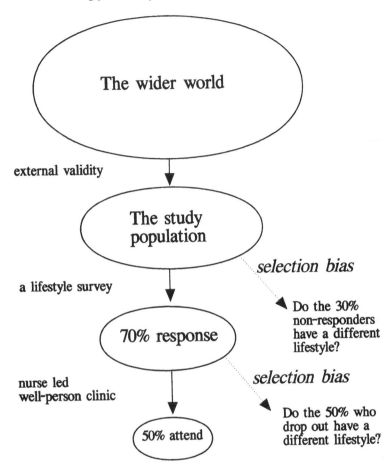

Figure 4.1 Selection bias: non-response and dropout.

advantage for the intervention is thus observed. The loss to follow-up has distorted the result. This is bias.

Selection bias is illustrated in Figure 4.1, showing a 70% response to a postal lifestyle survey, which is followed by a 50% response to an invitation to those who returned questionnaires to attend a 'well-person' clinic.

INFORMATION BIAS

Many of you reading the survey example above will have spotted another problem. Suppose that our lifestyle survey has a 90% response, and that a small study of non-responders has established that non-response will not have made much difference to the results.

There is no selection bias. However, there may be flaws in the questionnaire information itself, about smoking for example. In particular, smokers may systematically choose to underestimate their habit, whilst non-smokers classify themselves correctly. The proportion of non-smokers is inflated, and the nature and extent of smoking will be underestimated. This is an example of information bias.

Again there is a danger of mixing up bias within the study with issues of implication and external validity. If the purpose of the study were to compare the local prevalence of 'smoking as judged by a postal questionnaire' with the prevalence of smoking obtained from a national survey using an identical questionnaire, then information bias is not necessarily present. Like is being compared with like – even if the smoking information misrepresents the 'truth'. The truth in this example might, for example, be measured by 'smoking as judged by a chemical test which would establish the exact smoking levels during the past 24 hours'. Whether measurements in a study are biased or not depends on the objectives of the study.

Information bias, you will recall, can arise from the **instrument** used to obtain the information (this would be the questionnaire in the example above), from **patient error** in providing the information, or from **observer error** in obtaining the information. Such errors will be a source of bias if they distort the comparison between study groups.

> If, in the example above, local prevalence of smoking assessed by questionnaire is compared with a national study which used cotinine levels in the blood as a measure of smoking habits, then like is not being compared with like and a possible instrument bias has been introduced.
>
> If, in the trial of physical activity advice outlined above, the nurse was influenced in her questioning of the participants by her knowledge of whether they were in the intervention or control group, this will be a potential source of observer bias.

Information bias can affect both observational and intervention studies. Indeed much of the effort in designing intervention studies goes into separating the collection of information by observers from knowledge about who has had the intervention.

> In a trial to compare two drugs in primary care, the two drugs were made to appear identical. The patients who received the drug were unaware which preparation they were receiving.

Likewise the doctor carrying out the initial assessment did not know to which group each patient would be allocated and the nurse carrying out the follow-up interview to ascertain the outcome was similarly unaware. This procedure of **double blinding** (both subject and investigator unaware of the intervention) is designed to avoid the chance that knowledge of the intervention would influence symptom reporting by patients or the opinions of the clinical assessors. Information is thus kept free of bias.

Information bias related to the instrument used for measurement in a study can take different forms, and once again it is crucial to relate any judgement on bias to the objective of the study. Consider the three examples which follow.

1 During a survey of blood pressure in a practice it was discovered that one sphygmomanometer was giving erroneously high readings. Since a cut-off for diagnosing hypertension had been decided at the start of the study, this had led to over-diagnosis: a bias arising from instrument error.

2 In a survey of the need for knee replacement in a local population, a questionnaire about knee pain was used to identify subjects who might need knee replacement. It was pointed out to the researchers that radiographic knee osteoarthritis can often be advanced and disabling without causing pain, and also that much knee pain is not caused by osteoarthritis. So how useful is a questionnaire about knee pain? Of limited use in isolation is the short answer. However, it is important not to throw the baby out with the bath water. Knowing the prevalence of knee pain in the community might be a useful starting point.

3 A district health authority decided to start a morbidity register in practices with identical computer systems. There was interest locally in the possibility that certain urban areas had a higher prevalence of asthma than rural areas because of traffic pollution. Asthma diagnoses on computer were identified from two practices. Surprisingly, the rural practice had a much higher prevalence of asthma than the urban practice. On further investigation it was found that the rural practice employed clerical time to update morbidity records to ensure diagnoses were entered on the computer. In the urban practice 'we put a diagnosis on computer if we think about it, although unfortunately Jack doesn't believe in doing it anyway'.

All these problems of information bias can be dealt with in the study design and preparation. Sphygmomanometers can be calibrated at the start of a study, and checked systematically during the study. The relation between knee pain and other parameters, such as an X-ray, can be established in a small initial pilot study and the right 'case definition' for the particular study established. And Jack can be sent on a (long and intensive) training course to modify his values and beliefs about computerized morbidity information!

BIAS IN GENERALIZING: DO THE RESULTS APPLY OUTSIDE THE STUDY?

You are happy with the study so far – no obvious bias in the study design, internal validity OK.

Applying the result to the outside world involves external validity. The issue of bias raises its head again, and considering it is part of the process of critical reflection.

This will be dealt with in depth in Chapter 6, but some examples will illustrate two special issues.

'Intention to treat'

The idea that there is one sort of bias that directly distorts a study result and another sort that affects the way you generalize the result to the world outside is wrapped up in the approach to study analysis known as 'intention to treat'.

Example: weight reduction in hypertensives

A general practitioner sets up a study of weight reduction in the treatment of mild hypertension. He recruits a large number of mild hypertensives from a screening programme in the practice population. He invites all those who are over the average weight for their age and height to participate in a trial before drug treatment is considered. Some decline, most accept. Those who agree to take part are randomly allocated to receiving brief general 'coronary risk' advice about diet, smoking and physical activity, and arrangements are made to check their blood pressures every 2 months for 6 months. Patients in the other group receive the same brief GP advice, but in addition they attend a dietitian's clinic once every 2 weeks for 3 months to reduce weight, followed by monthly visits to 6 months.

At the 6-month point the GP manages to see all the patients in the trial to check their blood pressures. However, 50% of the weight reduction group had defaulted on their dietitian appointments, although half of those who turned up had actually managed to lose weight and to maintain that weight loss.

The results were as follows:

1 Modest overall falls in both blood pressure and weight were observed in both groups after 6 months. The mean changes were similar in the two groups.
2 Among the patients who declined to take part in the study mean blood pressure and weight were unchanged after 6 months.
3 In the diet group:
  a In those who defaulted from the dietitian's clinic there was no change in mean blood pressure or weight after 6 months.
  b In those who attended the dietitian throughout the 6 months but did not lose weight, there was no change in mean blood pressure.
  c In those who attended the dietician and lost weight, weight loss was associated with a fall in blood pressure.

All these results are in themselves legitimate. We might want to know more about the methods to be reassured that they were not biased. For example, did the nurse checking the blood pressures know to which group they belonged? Did the doctor reviewing the patients at 6 months know group membership?

Which of the results should the authors emphasize? If the first overall findings were given headline status, it might imply that offering dietitian appointments is worthless for reducing blood pressure. If the subgroup result 3c were emphasized, the conclusion might be that weight loss helps to reduce blood pressure.

The choice of result depends on the purpose of the study. If different criteria are applied to the two study groups to produce a comparison, then bias may creep in.

For example, if defaulters from the diet clinic are excluded from the results, the conclusion would be 'definite benefit for dietitian referral'. But like is not being compared with like – we have ignored one effect of referring to a dietitian: some patients will not comply, will dropout and will not lose weight. If the GP is asking the question 'What would happen if I brought in a dietitian for all the obese mild hypertensives?', this comparison would give an erroneous answer. It is a form of bias because of unequal dropout in the two intervention groups.

A more correct answer to the GP's practical question comes from the 'intention to treat' analysis. Everyone referred to the dietitian, irrespective of subsequent attendance or compliance, is compared with everyone given brief GP advice only, regardless also of their subsequent attendance. This stresses that dropout and poor compliance are important outcomes in themselves. Like is being compared with like except in the one aspect of interest to the GP: referral to a dietitian.

However, the GP-researcher may have a much more specific question – if a patient loses weight under dietitian supervision in general practice, will there be clinically important reductions in blood pressure? This is less pragmatic because it ignores the problems of dropout and the failure of so much weight reduction advice. However, it addresses an important point: if weight loss actually occurs, is it a worthwhile treatment of high blood pressure? For this question an 'explanatory' analysis, comparing controls with the subgroup who attend the dietitian and lose weight, is reasonable.

Jargon corner

Different types of study highlight the issues discussed above.

Efficacy: Does a treatment, procedure or intervention actually do what it is claimed to do? If a trial addresses this point, it is called 'explanatory'. External validity or generalizability is less important than internal validity.

Effectiveness: Here the question is broader – given an efficacious treatment or intervention, does it actually work in the real world, with all the non-compliance, refusals and exclusions? Pragmatic trials with 'intention to treat' analyses attempt to address such questions.

Efficiency: Even if an intervention is effective, is it as efficient (in terms of cost, labour and training, for example) as the alternatives? Cost-effectiveness and health economics studies address such questions.

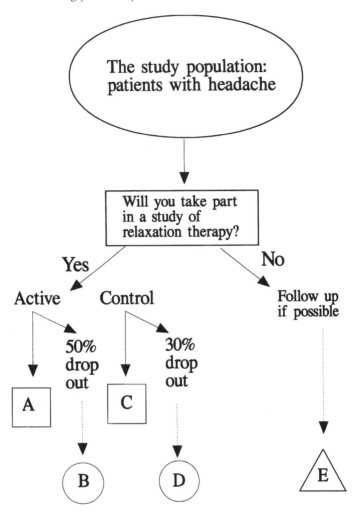

Figure 4.2 Different groups for analysis in a randomized controlled trial.

The difference between 'intention to treat' analysis and 'outcome-of-treatment' or 'explanatory' analysis is illustrated by an example in Figure 4.2: a trial of relaxation therapy in patients with headache. Some decline to take part in the study (group E), and there is a different dropout rate in the two arms of the trial (group B are the 50% who drop out from the group receiving active therapy; group D are the 30% who drop out from the control group). Let us assume that outcome in those who remain in the trial is measured at 6 months, and that some outcome data are obtained from the groups who dropped out or who did not wish to take part in the study. Possible analyses include:

1 Ideal intention-to-treat analysis = outcome (A + B) vs outcome (C + D) vs outcome (E)
2 Usual intention-to-treat analysis = outcome (A + B) vs outcome (C + D)
3 Outcome-of-treatment analysis = outcome (A) vs outcome (C)

Confounding

You have searched the methods and the data, and you have decided that the authors have dealt with possible bias internal to the study. You are considering whether the results justify the conclusions and something doesn't seem quite right. You wonder whether there could be a different explanation for the results than the one put forward by the authors.

TEST YOURSELF: CONFOUNDING

In the National Morbidity Survey in General Practice (Royal College of General Practitioners, 1995) variations in the incidence of consultations for sinusitis were found between different areas of the country, as well as a higher incidence in non-manual social classes. One interpretation is that living in low-lying areas of the country or working in factory atmospheres are risks for sinusitis.

Question

What alternative explanations might there be? Write down your thoughts before reading on.

Suggested answers

1 One doctor's sinusitis is another's cold. The diagnosis written down by the doctor is the label they choose to use. Regional differences may reflect different labelling habits. If you were using the data to investigate the theory that low-lying areas have more sinusitis than hilly areas, this would need to be taken into account.

2 One influence on the diagnostic label might be the patient's social status. More highly educated patients may use the terms 'sinusitis' in presenting their symptoms; it may be used by the doctor as meaning 'this is a patient with a bad cold to whom I am going to give an antibiotic'.

Studies of the relationship between sinusitis and factors such as geography or social class may be open to such **confounding** by diagnostic behaviour – diagnosis varies with doctor and with social class, and this variation provides an alternative explanation of the differences in the study.

These alternative explanations are known as **confounders**. The boundary between confounding and information bias is a thin one, and you do not need to spend hours agonizing over it. A more traditional example will highlight the difference.

> In a study of lifestyle and cancer, coffee drinkers had more lung cancer than non-coffee drinkers. Perhaps coffee is carcinogenic. But perhaps coffee drinkers smoke more cigarettes than those who do not drink coffee. When non-smokers and smokers were later analysed separately, there was no relationship between lung cancer and coffee drinking habits.
>
> If information about coffee drinking had been collected in different ways in those with and without lung cancer, you might have worried that the result was suspect – that there was information bias.
>
> You are happy with the result of the study but you also accept the analysis that the apparent link between coffee drinking and lung cancer could all be explained by smoking. Here smoking is a confounder.

The great advantage of randomized controlled trials is that they get rid of confounding. Age, sex, social class, previous diet and smoking, for example, are all features which may affect the way in which blood pressure responds to dietary changes. If patients entering a trial of weight reduction to reduce their blood pressure are allocated at random to the intervention or control group, then on average (as the numbers build up) the groups will balance out with respect to such potential confounders. What is more, they will balance with respect to confounders the researchers do not know about or have not measured. Differences in outcome can more confidently be ascribed to the one remaining distinction between the groups – whether they had the intervention or not.

Example: aspirin and acute myocardial infarction

There have been a number of randomized controlled trials of the effect on mortality of aspirin taken early after an acute myocardial infarction (NHS Centre for Reviews and Dissemination, 1995). There are many influences on the outcome of myocardial infarction and it can be imagined how these same factors might also influence the likelihood of receiving aspirin – the age of the patient, the proximity of the hospital, the presence of heart failure. So the idea of randomly allocating patients to receive aspirin or not in a trial ensures that the groups being compared are alike in all characteristics except for the fact that one group received aspirin and the other group a placebo.

Jargon corner

Confounding: The other explanation

A confounder (e.g. age) is related to both the outcome (e.g. death after a myocardial infarction) and the presumed cause or intervention being studied (e.g. years of cigarette smoking or previous use of aspirin).

The most effective approach to confounding is randomization in intervention studies. In observational studies, the effects of known confounders can be analysed by specific statistical methods.

The principle of confounding is illustrated in another example in Figure 4.3. Consider two towns: Oldtown is a well-off retirement town on the South Coast of England; Youngtown is a relatively poor northern industrial city. The incidence of coronary heart disease (CHD) in Oldtown is higher than in Youngtown. Given the well-known link between CHD and the less well-off socioeconomic

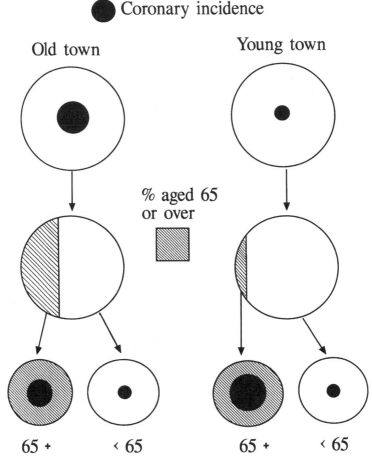

Figure 4.3 An example of confounding.

groups, why should this be? The answer is that a confounding factor (age) is powerfully associated with CHD incidence, and the average age of Oldtown is higher than that of Youngtown. If we stratify the two towns by age, using a cutoff of 65 years for example, we see that CHD incidence is actually lower in 65 year olds in Oldtown than among 65 year olds in Youngtown, and furthermore is lower in those under 65 in Oldtown than similarly aged people in Youngtown. This fits with the known distribution of CHD according to socioeconomic circumstances. The paradox arose because CHD incidence is much higher above 65 years than below 65, and Oldtown had proportionately more old people than Youngtown.

Age is a confounder here because it is strongly related to the disease (CHD) and to the factor being studied (residence in Oldtown or Youngtown).

TEST YOURSELF: CONFOUNDING

You compare the prevalence of diabetes in your practice population with that in a colleague's practice in another part of the country. They are different.

Question

Before you conclude that this represents a geographical difference in occurrence rates, what other explanations would you consider?

Suggested answer

Think in terms of three headings.

Bias: Information bias: Different definitions of diabetes in the two practices.
Selection bias: Variations in the completeness of diabetic registers for example.

Confounding: Differences in age and social class between the two populations might be the explanation of any differences.

Chance variation: How many cases were compared, and how large are the two practice populations?

Summary box

Bias: any aspect of a study which might systematically distort the true result. For example, patients in the active treatment group of a randomized controlled trial appear to do better because those who develop side-effects drop out from the study.

Bias can broadly be classified into two types: **selection** and **information** bias.

TEST YOURSELF: STUDY DESIGN

DIET AND NEURAL TUBE DEFECTS

Questions

1 A geographical variation around Britain in the occurrence of congenital neural tube defects has been observed. One interpretation is that this pattern reflects regional variations in diet among conceiving mothers. Think of some potential confounders of this explanation.

2 The idea is put forward that, if a woman takes vitamin supplements at the time of conception, the fetus is protected against neural tube defects.

   A study is mounted to test this idea. Mothers of children with a neural tube defect are asked whether they would be willing to be interviewed: there is a 70% response. They are asked to recall their use of vitamin supplements during conception. A sample of mothers of normal children are invited to act as controls and to have an identical interview: in this group there is a 95% response. No difference is found between the two groups with respect to vitamin supplementation at conception.

   a What sort of study is this?
   b What biases might be important in this study?

3 A group of women who have already had one child with a neural tube defect and who are planning a further pregnancy are invited to take part in a study to follow the outcome of their next pregnancy. Within this group, women who report that they regularly take vitamin supplementation are to be compared with women who do not routinely take vitamins. Follow-up is 95% in both groups. In the subsequent pregnancies the incidence of neural tube defects among the children is shown in Table 4.1, taken from Smithells *et al.* (1980):

   a What type of study is this?
   b What advantages does this study have over the study in question 2?
   What are the problems with this study?
   c What further study would you do?

4 A group of women who have previously had an affected pregnancy agree to take part in a study in which they will either

Table 4.1 Number of pregnancies by outcome and vitamin supplementation

	Vitamin supplementation	
	Yes	*No*
Neural tube defects	1	13
No neural tube defects	178	260

Table 4.2 Numbers of pregnancies by outcome and vitamin supplementation

	Intervention	
	Vitamin	*Placebo*
Neural tube defects	6	21
No neural tube defects	593	602

take a multivitamin supplement regularly during the time in which they plan to conceive and during any subsequent pregnancy, or they will take a placebo tablet in identical fashion. The group to which they are allocated is determined by a randomization procedure. The results are shown in Table 4.2, taken from reference MCR Vitamin Study Research Group (1991):

a What sort of study is this?
b What are the advantages compared with the study in in question 3? What are the disadvantages?
b Is the difference between this result and the result from question 3 important?

Suggested answers

1 Poor diet is being linked to neural tube defects because of geographical variation in occurrence of these problems. This is one explanation, but there are clearly many alternative possibil-

ities or confounders of the diet idea. For example, smoking, environmental pollution, and parental ill-health all vary geographically and all may influence the occurrence of neural tube defects.

2 a This study is observational, retrospective and controlled.

  b Selection: the poorer response in mothers with affected children might be important if, for example, non-responders were more likely to be those mothers who had not taken vitamins.

    Information: recall of vitamin supplements at time of conception might be poor; if it were poor in both groups it might not matter, although important differences might be blurred or hidden; more important might be the influence that having a child with a neural tube defect has on recall of events at the time of conception.

3 a This study is observational, prospective and controlled.

  b Because this study does not depend on recall of events after the birth and because follow-up was good in both groups, bias and internal validity would seem to be less of a problem than in the previous study. However, it seems highly likely that women who choose to take regular vitamin supplements and those who do not are likely to differ in many other ways which themselves might influence the likelihood of a further complicated pregnancy (e.g. age, smoking, physical fitness, other aspects of diet). In other words, potential confounders are likely to be thick on the ground.

  c The obvious way round the confounder issue would be to do a randomized controlled trial.

4 a A randomized controlled prospective intervention study.

  b The advantage is that confounders should balance out between the two groups. Disadvantages would include: (i) How many women would actually agree to take part in the study – if very few, would it have any external validity? (ii) What of the ethics of such a study, given the large beneficial effect seen in the earlier observational study even if it was flawed by possible confounding? (iii) Could the result be extrapolated to women who had not yet had an affected pregnancy?

  c Both studies suggest a protective effect of peri-conceptual vitamin supplementation. The fact that the effect was stronger in the observational study suggests that confounding was important. However, the confounding did not explain away a direct effect of vitamins, as evidenced by the intervention study.

DO PATIENTS READ HEALTH PROMOTION POSTERS?

Question

Write short comments on the methods in this study, listing good points and problem points.

Title: Do patients read health promotion posters in the waiting room? A study in one general practice (Ward, 1994).

Summary
Background: General practitioners are aware of the need to provide easily accessible health promotion information for their patients. Although many practices use health promotion posters in their surgeries, there appears to have been no formal evaluation of their effectiveness.

Aim: A study was undertaken to investigate whether patients read and remembered waiting room posters, and if so, what factors influenced this.

Method: A short questionnaire was distributed to patients in one practice following their consultation. It asked what they remembered of the poster display in the waiting room.

Results: Of 319 patients attending a doctor during the study period 82% said they had noticed the posters, 95% of whom reported they had also read them. Patients over 50 years of age were significantly more likely to say they had read the posters than younger patients, but significantly fewer showed interest in further information. The sex of patients did not influence their reading of posters or their interest in further health promotion literature. The longer patients had to wait for the doctor, the more likely they were to remember the subject of the posters correctly. Some subjects appeared to attract more patients' attention than others, in particular the displays about smoking cessation and about the human immunodeficiency virus (HIV) and the acquired immune deficiency syndrome (AIDS). Overall 53% said they would be interested in more information.

Conclusion: Patients say they read and remember the subject of waiting room posters. Posters in the waiting room can increase awareness of health promotion issues.

Methods in full: The waiting room notice boards chosen for the study were covered with bright blue card. Other health promotion material in the room was removed. The display was made up of posters selected from the local health promotion unit in Manchester, and supplemented with handmade stencilled headings. Four topics were chosen on a rotating monthly basis: healthy eating, smoking cessation, alcohol reduction, and information about the human immunodeficiency virus (HIV) and AIDS.

Patients were excluded from the study if they were under 16 years old, or attending with another person, or had already been entered into the study. At the end of each consultation, the doctor gave patients a short questionnaire asking them what they remembered about the display and how long they had waited to be seen. The questionnaire was quick and easy to complete. It was filled in by patients at a table in the hall, and then left in a box near the exit. The layout of the surgery was such that patients left the building after seeing the doctor without re-entering the waiting room where the posters were displayed. The patients were not prevented from reviewing the poster display although it would have taken them out of their way to do so. The survey was conducted by two out of five of the doctors at any one time during the first week of each new poster display in order to avoid congestion in the corridors. Interim analysis indicated that the first display, on healthy eating, was noticed more than subsequent displays. To see if this was a result of a 'new look' effect in the waiting room, the same display was repeated at the end of the study, hence there were five study weeks.

The age–sex distribution of the sample was compared with that of a typical week's surgery to ascertain if the sample was representative of the population of patients using the practice. Results were analysed using *SPSSPC+* in order to calculate frequencies and chi-square tests.

Suggested answers

Good points

Avoiding information bias

a A mix of posters was used, with one display used twice to rule out a novelty effect.
b Attempts were made to avoid patients seeing the posters after they had been given the questionnaire.

Making it practical

a The study ensured corridors were not congested and the surgery visit was not uncomfortable for patients.

Avoiding selection bias

a There were sensible exclusions such as attendance with another person or previous participation in the study.
b The representativeness of the sample was checked by comparing its age and sex distribution with a 'typical' week of attenders.

Problem points

Presentation of methods

a Some details have been left out or are vague.

Selection

a Poorly described.
b 'Two out of five doctors at any one time' – was this arranged in a formal rotation? Were all patients in the relevant surgeries asked to participate?
c Was the study anonymous or could non-participants be identified? (This would be useful if a response rate were to be calculated and attempts made to investigate whether non-responders were different in important ways to participants.)

Information

a Content and validity of the questionnaire are poorly described.
b Is recall of waiting time a reliable measure? This could have been validated in one surgery against actual wait, or measured independently in everyone.
c What questions were actually asked? It is reasonable to expect such detail if it is a new questionnaire, particularly if it is a short one.
d Were questions about the posters 'open-ended' or 'closed'?

Chance variation

a No justification of sample size is given.

REFERENCES

Kopec, J.A., and Esdalle, J.M. (1990). Bias in case-control studies. A review. *Journal of Epidemiology and Community Health*, **44**, 179–86.

MRC Vitamin Study Research Group. (1991). Prevention of neural tube defects: results of the Medical Research Council Vitamin Study. *Lancet*, **333**, 131–7.

NHS Centre for Reviews and Dissemination. (1995). Aspirin and myocardial infarction. *Effectiveness Matters*, **1**. University of York.

Royal College of General Practitioners and Office of National Statistics. (1995). *Morbidity studies in a general practice* 1981–1982. London: HMSO

Sackett D.L. (1979). Bias in analytic research. *Journal of Chronic Diseases*, **32**, 51–63.

Smithells, R.W., Sheppard, S., Schorah, C.J., Seller, M.J., Nevin, N.C., Harris, R., Read, A.P., and Fielding, D.W. (1980). Possible prevention of neural-tube defects by periconceptional vitamin supplementation. *Lancet*, **1**, 339–40.

Ward, K., and Hawthorne, K. (1994). Do patients read health promotion posters in the waiting room? A study in one general practice. *British Journal of General Practice*, **44**, 583–5.

5

Do I understand the results? Statistics

Statistics has got a bad name with health professionals. The thought of P values and chi-square tests is enough to make most of us quake. Why does this branch of medical science evoke such terror? How has it come to exert such power?

The randomized controlled trial or the 'RCT', the Rolls Royce of study design, is the nearest we get in clinical or health-related research to the classical scientific experiment. Because we cannot tightly control every aspect of experiments involving humans, the randomized trial offers an alternative. Instead of keeping all possible confounding factors constant, randomization is an attempt to allocate them reasonably equally between the experimental groups. Differences between the groups can then be attributed either to the one thing which is systematically different between the groups (i.e. the intervention) or to the probability that the differences arose by chance in the course of randomization. Probability statistics estimate the latter, but their influence has extended into the whole medical literature, and statistical tests of 'significance' (embodied in the 'P' value) have been used as a judgement on the truth or otherwise of a study result.

This iron grip of the 'P' value is now loosening, and it is statisticians themselves who lead the assault on its indiscriminate and incorrect application in judging truth in medical research. Medical statisticians are more concerned with study design (how to reduce bias and confounding) than with statistical tests of probability alone. The most important statistics are those which are used to summarize data which is measured or counted (quantitative data).

There are three main types of quantitative data:

1 Data measured on a numerical or 'continuous' scale (e.g. height, weight, haemoglobin).
2 Data in separate categories (e.g. smoker/ non-smoker; male/ female).
3 Ranked data which applies a rank order to categorical or numerical data (e.g. recovered, improved, no different, worse).

Such data need summarizing to characterize a study group. For categorical data, the proportion or percentage in each group is one obvious way of summarizing the result. For continuous data other solutions have to be found.

SUMMARIZING THE DATA

The statistician's favourite distribution of continuous data is the normal or Gaussian distribution (illustrated in Fig. 5.1) and much time is spent trying to get data to correspond to this distribution, because it has all sorts of useful properties. It is familiar because many distributions follow the general principle that most people fall

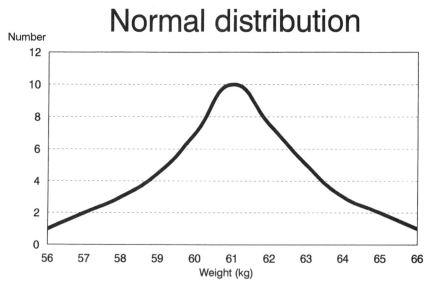

Figure 5.1 The normal distribution.

in the middle and as you go to the extremes in both directions so there are fewer people.

Your research project: find the weight of the average British nurse

In order to obtain this crucial information, you set out to find a sample of nurses. With your measuring scales in one hand and personal computer in the other, you visit your local District General Hospital and are lucky enough to find 47 volunteers who are prepared to be weighed. You jot down the 47 weights and head back to the laboratory. Although statisticians often give the opposite impression, the main task of statistics is to make life simpler. To make life simpler, it would be nice to summarize three aspects of your data. You will need:

1 An average weight for your sample.
2 A measure of how the individual values are dispersed about the average.
3 Information about whether the distribution is normal or not.

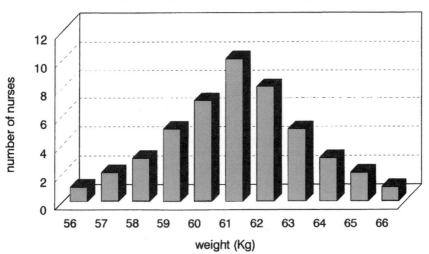

Figure 5.2 A histogram showing the frequency distribution of different weight categories.

You start by drawing a histogram or bar diagram of your results, as shown in Figure 5.2. Along the horizontal axis you plot weight in kilograms and along the vertical axis you plot the number of nurses with any given weight.

The next thing to do is to find the average: a statistician would call this the 'central tendency'. There are three sorts of average:

- **Arithmetic mean**: the sum of the individual weights divided by the number of nurses
- **Median**: the mid-point value in your sample series when they are ranked in ascending order
- **Mode**: the commonest value in your sample

In our example, the arithmetic mean, the median and mode are exactly the same, 61 kg. This is a good indicator that the distribution is normal.

Sometimes data form a **skewed distribution** in which there are some extreme values which pull the data to one end of the distribution.

In Figure 5.3 the tops of the histogram bars have been joined together to form a frequency distribution and once again the

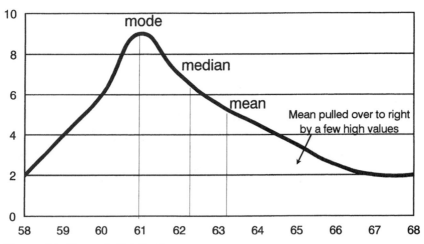

Figure 5.3 Skewed distribution

number of nurses is represented on the vertical axis and weight is the variable along the horizontal axis. This shows that the mode, median and mean do **not** coincide in a skewed distribution.

There is a 'tail' to the curve which means that there were a small number of rather heavy nurses in the sample obtained. Look at the effect which this has on the mean. The very heavy nurses influence the mean, 'pulling it over' towards the heavier values.

Let's use another simple example to illustrate this point.

Consider the series of numbers 1, 2, 3, 4, 5. Add them all up and you get 15. Divide 15 by 5 to find the average and the answer is 3. Now consider the series 1, 2, 3, 4, 90. Add them all up and you get 100. Divide by 5 (the number of items) to get the average which is now 20. The simple substitution of a single extreme value (90) for the last item has increased the arithmetic mean from 3 to 20. In this sort of situation the **median value** is useful. Remember that the median is the one in the middle so in the series 1, 2, 3, 4, 5 the item 3 is the one in the middle, flanked by the 1 and the 2 on the one hand and the 4 and the 5 on the other. In the second series 1, 2, 3, 4, 90, the item in the middle is still 3 flanked by the 1 and the 2 before it and 4 and the 90 after it. Statisticians would therefore argue that the median is a better measure of central tendency in this sort of situation.

Such skewed distributions are quite common in research papers these days with the focus on health care (days in hospital after a procedure, practice variations in numbers of night calls) and the use of ranked data for self-rating questionnaires. Although the mean can be used even when the distribution deviates quite a way from the ideal 'normal', it is always useful to look for the median.

For those of you who are beginning to feel anxious about statistics beyond the summarizing stuff, you may wish to turn to the section headed 'Has the right statistical test been chosen?' (p.109).

Measures of dispersion

The simplest way of summarizing how much variation there is within the sample is to quote the **range** from the smallest to the largest value. Unfortunately this is easily influenced by one or two extreme values. Consider the series of numbers 1, 2, 3, 4, 5. The

Normal distribution

2 curves with same mean but different dispersion

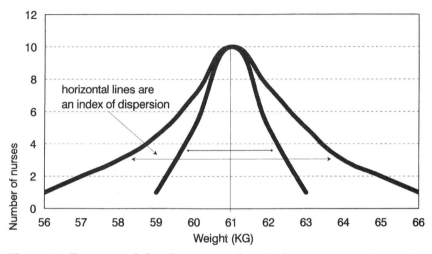

Figure 5.4 Two normal distributions, each with the same mean, but with a different spread of values.

range is 4. Now consider the series 1, 2, 3, 4, 90. The range has increased to 89 purely because of the one extreme value at the end of the series. For this reason more sophisticated measures of dispersion are used.

Consider Figure 5.4. Both distributions have the same mean but they are obviously very different. The distribution on the inside has very little variation. If this were a sample of nurses, the weights of all the nurses would be close to the mean. In the outside distribution, there is much more variation. There are a few very light nurses and also a few very heavy nurses with a 'normal' spread of nurses in between. What we need is a measure to give us a guide to the width of the main part of these curves.

A simple method is to average out all the deviations from the mean. In the example given, the weight of each nurse would be compared with the mean and the deviation from the mean calculated. Then the total of all the deviations in the sample would be added up and divided by 47, the number of nurses within the sample. The result is the average or **mean deviation**.

The **standard deviation** (SD) is a very similar index of the width of the curve and a good guide to the amount of variation within the sample. Unless you have a particular interest in statistics, you do not really need to know how it is calculated.

One of the reasons that statisticians prefer to use the standard deviation is because it relates to the special properties of the normal distribution curve. Whatever the scale being used, if values are normally distributed, the mean plus or minus one standard deviation will always include 68% of the data. More importantly, the mean plus or minus two standard deviations will include approximately 95% of the data with only 2.5% above and 2.5% below this range. Statistics related to this distribution are referred to as **parametric statistics**.

This is an important concept. With reference to our sample of 47 nurses, if the sample has a normal distribution and if one measures the weight of any nurse chosen at random from the sample, there is a 95% chance that the nurse chosen will have a weight which lies within the range 'mean plus or minus two standard deviations'. This is summarized in Figure 5.5.

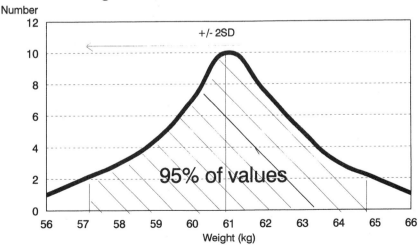

Figure 5.5 Normal distribution.

Dispersion can be summarized for non-normal distributions as well. One way of doing this when the median is used is to indicate two further points on the distribution: the value below which 25% of the readings lie and the value below which 75% of the values lie. These points will obviously lie each to one side of the median and they represent the '**interquartile range**'. This range is the appropriate measure of dispersion to accompany the median and once again guards against the distortion that outliers may give to a summary based on the full range of observations.

ESTIMATING THE EFFECT OF CHANCE

The next concept is probably the most difficult for non-statisticians to grasp. So don't worry if it doesn't make sense immediately. While considering your research project, your supervisor decides that finding the weight of the average British nurse is not a challenging enough task and now you must consider a more complex issue: Are doctors heavier than nurses? In order to answer this question you take a similar sample of doctors and measure their weight. On this occasion you find that the mean weight of 47 doctors is 66 kg compared with the mean weight of the nurses at 61 kg. But is there a **real** difference between the groups?

There are two ways in which a difference in the weights of doctors and nurses may appear which does not represent a true difference:

1 The way in which we have selected our groups may be different: for example, an advert on a notice-board may have missed the heaviest nurses, who may be self-conscious about being weighed, whereas a random questionnaire to the doctors might have included the full range. Statistics cannot compensate for such **selection bias**.
2 If we are happy that each group is reasonably selected, have we by chance picked a light group of nurses and a heavy group of doctors? Statistics can help us here by allowing us to estimate the possible effects of chance variation on the results of any particular study. Assuming our sample is not biased, what we

wish to assess is how representative our small sample is likely to be of all doctors and nurses working in Britain. Whether each group is representative is assessed by the **sampling error**. If there is little sampling error the means will be accurate. If a new sample were taken the new mean would be similar to the original sample mean.

The **standard error of the mean** (SEM) is the way in which this is done. It is calculated by dividing the standard deviation by the square root of the number in the sample. This makes intuitive sense. If the standard deviation is large, this implies that there is a lot of variation within the sample, and this implies that there is likely to be a large amount of variation in the whole population. There is therefore more room for error in the mean. Sample size is important and in general the larger the sample, the more accurate the mean will be. But there is a sods law of statistics in this. The problem is that in order to double the accuracy of the mean one has to quadruple the size of the sample. This explains the square root sign in the following formula.

$$SEM = SD/\sqrt{n}$$

where n is the number in the sample. Note that the SEM is always smaller than the SD because it is calculated by dividing the SD by something.

The standard error of the mean can be used to define the **95% confidence interval for the mean**. If one were to take any other group of 47 nurses and calculate their mean weight, there is a 95% chance that the new mean obtained would lie in the range 'original mean plus or minus 2 SEM'.

The null hypothesis

Statisticians are not particularly helpful at this point because they introduce a new bit of jargon called the null hypothesis. The **null hypothesis** makes one assume that the difference observed between the two samples is simply due to random variation.

Jargon corner

Null hypothesis

There is a difference observed between two groups in a randomized trial. The null hypothesis then proposes 'suppose there is actually no difference between the two groups' and this leads to the question 'what then is the probability that this observed difference could have arisen by chance, during randomization?'.

95% confidence interval of the difference

There is a difference observed between two groups in a randomized trial. We can be 95% confident that the true difference between the groups, assuming no bias and efficient randomization, lies within the interval.

The next stage is to estimate the variation you would anticipate in random samples by using the standard error of the mean. Then you compare the differences you have actually observed between the samples with the predicted variation due to sampling error. If the differences observed are large and the predicted sampling error small then you reject the null hypothesis and say how unlikely it is. If that seems an upside down way of doing things, it probably is. Don't worry about it if you don't understand it. In practice what the critical reader does is:

1 Look at the actual difference between the means.
2 Look at the 95% confidence intervals to get a feel of the likely range of values which chance variation in samples of this size might give rise to.
3 Examine the probability value to see if the differences are more or less likely to have arisen by chance in this particular case.

In the example about doctors and nurses the standard deviation of each sample is about 2 kg and the standard error of the mean is less than 1 kg. The difference between the two means is 5 kg and its 95% confidence interval is 4–6 kg. So we interpret this by saying that we can be 95% confident that repeated samples of this size would have produced a range of mean differences between nurses and doctors of 4–6 kg. Chance cannot explain away the difference. But note that you have to make additional important judgements, separate to the issue of chance, as to whether this size of difference is important ('clinically significant') and to what extent it might have arisen because of study bias.

A 'P value' summarizes the probability that the point of 'no difference' or 'null point' has fallen within the 95% confidence interval of the observed difference (P is more than 5%: the difference is not significant statistically) or outside it (P is less than 5%: the observed difference is regarded as statistically significant). For normally distributed data, a *t* test is the statistical calculation which provides the P value.

What you may need to know about probability values

A *P* of 1.0 means there is a 100% chance that the difference observed between samples is simply due to random variation.

A *P* of 0.1 means there is a 10% chance that the difference observed is due to random variation.

A probability value of 0.05 means there is a 1 in 20 or 5% chance that the difference observed is simply due to sampling error. This is the conventionally accepted limit of statistical significance. Make sure you look carefully at the less than or greater than signs.

If *P* is greater than 0.05 the result is not statistically significant. If *P* is less than 0.05 it is statistically significant.

This is all 'convention' though and is not telling you the truth or the real significance of the result. The most important results to look at are the actual figures and their 95% confidence intervals. This helps you to ask first whether this difference is likely to be important (never mind its statistical significance), and whether the possible influence of chance as judged by the 95% confidence interval is likely to diminish that importance.

Jargon corner

Parametric statistics

These relate to data which:

1 are measured on a numerical scale;
2 have a normal distribution.

- The **mean** is the average: the measure of the centre of a normal distribution.
- The **standard deviation** is a summary measure of the dispersion of observed values about the mean in a normal distribution.
- The **standard** or **sampling error of the mean** is an index of the accuracy or precision of the mean in the sample under study.
- **95% confidence interval**: the range of values for a summary of sample data, such as a mean, which expresses the chance variation which arises from any random sampling. We can be 95% confident that the 'target population' value is contained within that range.

Statistics are not a guarantee of truth. They summarize the data. Data must first be examined for any bias. Then statistics can be used to summarize the likely effects of chance on the observed result.

CATEGORICAL DATA

Frequencies and proportions

The principles described above can be applied to categorical data. For example, suppose you decide to summarize the weights of the nurses by separating them into two categories: 62 kg and above, and less than 62 kg. There are 33 nurses who fall into the lighter group, summarized by a percentage (70%) or a proportion (0.7). From the sample size and the proportion itself, a standard error for the proportion can be calculated and hence a 95% confidence interval.

In a sample of 47 nurses, 70% were observed to be less than 62 kg in weight. If this were a random sample of nurses, we can be 95% confident that the proportion of all nurses who weigh less than 62 kg lies between 57% and 83%.

A bigger sample size would narrow this confidence interval.

The equivalent of a *t* test for categorical data is the **chi-square** test. Statistical textbooks give formulae for calculating this statistic based on frequencies, and the *P* value is looked up in chi-square tables. Again the same interpretation using 95% confidence intervals can be used as explained above.

> In the sample of 47 doctors, there are 24 who fall in the lighter group (less than 62 kg), i.e. 51%. For a sample of this size, the 95% confidence interval of this proportion is 37% to 65%, i.e. if this was a random sample of all doctors we would be 95% confident that the proportion of all doctors who weighed less than 62 kg lies between these two figures.

We may then wish to compare these two proportions (nurses vs doctors). Once again we must be very cautious about what we are comparing – there may be more male doctors than male nurses and doctors on average might be older than nurses, so any overall weight difference may be explained by the effects which age and gender have on weight. However, if these factors are taken account of and we have random samples of nurses and doctors, then it is legitimate to ask if the difference in weight between them might simply be due to chance variation in the two samples.

> The 95% confidence intervals of the two observed proportions overlap. In other words the difference in the proportions of doctors and nurses weighing less than 62 kg is not statistically significant.

Ranks and skewed data

Let us suppose that we were interested in the heights of the nurses and doctors but did not have a method to measure them. We put them altogether and stand them in a line in order of their 'eyeballed' height. Each gets a rank number from tallest to shortest. The question now is whether nurses tend to be shorter than doctors. This can be done by comparing the rankings of all the nurses with those of the doctors.

Note that the actual heights are not being used in this comparison, nor the actual proportion of nurses or doctors above a particular height: simply their position in a pecking order relative to each other. Where there is no measurement or distribution of measurement, the statistical methods of comparison are called 'non-parametric'. There are various methods available – rank order is only one. They are particularly relevant for skewed data, where the median is being used as the method of summary.

Jargon corner

Median: 50% of values are below it, useful for skewed distributions.

Interquartile range (IQR): measure of dispersion of observed values around a median (25% of values are below the lower end of the IQR, 25% above the upper end).

HOW IMPORTANT ARE STATISTICS TO THE CRITICAL READER?

Statistics are not as important as knowledge of study design issues and bias and confounding, and common sense. But critical readers may get weary of the 'do not worry about statistics' advice when they see them everywhere. Our brief review should be supplemented by good short textbooks, such as those of Campbell and Machin (1993) and Coggon (1995), if you are interested in tackling statistical issues in more detail.

Summary

- Statistics cannot tell us the truth.
- Statistics cannot solve a flaw in study design: if the study is biased, a bigger sample size simply increases the effect of the bias, even if the result becomes 'statistically significant'.
- If you are happy with the design, then in certain studies (particularly RCTs), statistics can help to evaluate the likely influence of chance on the result.
- The main role of statistics is to summarize data.

HAS THE RIGHT STATISTICAL TEST BEEN CHOSEN?

A quick guide for the critical reader.

Assuming you are happy with the validity of the data.

STEP 1: What sort of data is it and did they really need that test? Continuous, categorical or ranked?

STEP 2: If it is continuous data.
Is it normally distributed?
If yes:

- means and standard deviations describe the sample and its dispersion;
- the mean and the 95% confidence interval of the mean give a summary of the likely random error in the sampling;
- *t* tests might be used to calculate a *P* value if comparisons are being made.

If no:

- the median should be used as a summary, particularly if the data show it to be very different from the mean;
- the interquartile range summarizes the dispersion of the data;
- non-parametric statistical tests can be used.

STEP 3: If it is categorical data,

- summarized as a proportion or percentage. 95% confidence intervals to indicate the influence of sampling error can be shown.
- chi-square tests can be used to calculate *P* values for data displayed as counts or frequencies.
- non-parametric tests can be used for ranked data.

Figure 5.6 illustrates some of the basic choices and routes to go down when choosing a statistical test.

SUMMARIZING EFFECTS AND ASSOCIATIONS

Much medical research investigates links between treatment and cure, and between risk and disease. Any comparison between one

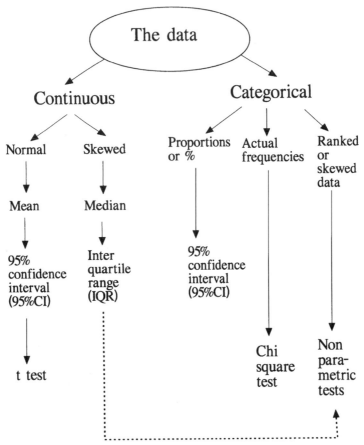

Figure 5.6 Some basic choices of statistical tests.

group and a control group is an investigation of the association between cause and effect.

For example:

- In a randomized trial of consultation style, we are interested in the association between the style and the outcome in each of the trial groups.
- In a study of coronary heart disease and physical activity we are interested in whether different frequencies of heart attacks occur in association with particular types of activity.
- In a study of a new test for otitis media we are interested in the association between positive results gathered by the new test and results obtained at operation.

One simple way of expressing an association is to calculate the difference between the summary statistics (means, medians or proportions) for each comparison group.

For example:

- The mean weight of British doctors was 2 kg higher than the mean weight of British nurses.
- The proportion of people stating that they smoked was 25% in the North of England compared with 15% in the South.

There are, however, some specific measures of association.

Some helpful words

Ratio: any number (numerator) divided by another (denominator).

Proportion: a ratio in which the denominator contains the numerator 'the proportion of men in Britain who smoke is 15%, i.e. out of every 100 men in Britain there are 15 who smoke'. A **risk** is a proportion with a time element added. In 1 year the risk of an adult developing a new episode of shoulder pain is 1 in 100, i.e. out of every 100 adults at the start of a year, there will be one who, during the year, will develop shoulder pain.

Odds: a ratio in which the denominator does not include the numerator. The odds of a British male smoking are 15:85 – for every 85 men who do not smoke, there are 15 who do.

Risk ratio: this is one risk divided by another. So the 1-year risk of a new episode of shoulder pain in those aged 45 years and over is twice the 1-year risk in those aged below 45, a risk ratio of 2. This is one way to measure the **association** between age and shoulder pain.

Odds ratio: this is one odds divided by another. So the odds of a British man smoking (15:85) are more than twice as high as the odds of a British woman smoking (10:90), an odds ratio of 2.5. The odds ratio has become increasingly popular as a measure of association in published studies. This despite its being intuitively more difficult to grasp than a risk ratio. The reason for its popularity is that it has some interesting properties. For example, you can calculate the odds ratio when essential information to calculate risk ratios is missing. New statistical packages on computer often calculate the odds ratio directly using a technique called logistic regression, which allows confounders of the main association to be taken into account in the analysis. For example, the odds ratio for the association between contraceptive pill use and deep venous thrombosis in women is 3.0, after adjusting for the possible influence of age and weight.

> *Question*: If the odds ratio for the link between active consultation style and patient satisfaction is 2, how would you interpret this?

> *Answer*: The likelihood of patients having a high satisfaction score given an active consultation was twice as high as having a high satisfaction score given a passive style of consultation.

Odds ratios and risk ratios allow associations to be summarized.

Even more helpful words

Imagine you are faced with a patient who smokes and wishes to know about the risks of smoking. You might put it to him as a risk ratio:

> 'As a smoker, you are 7 times more likely than a non-smoker to die of lung cancer'

Sounds impressive. However your patient is a bit of a mathematician, and puts a question back to you.

> 'Ah, but how likely is a non-smoker to die of lung cancer?'

You stifle the urge to complete the circle by replying 'seven times less likely than a smoker'. Your patient wants to know more: the actual risk of dying of lung cancer, not a relative statement such as '7 times more than . . .'.

Here things get a little complicated because there may be no data to hand which apply to your particular patient. But we can turn to a published UK study, which has been a major source of evidence on the health risks of smoking. It is a prospective observational study of British doctors who were recruited to the study more than 40 years ago (Doll, 1976). Lung cancer mortality in the doctors' study showed:

- 49 deaths per 100 000 smokers per year;
- 7 deaths per 100 000 non-smokers per year.

The risk ratio is clearly 7. But we can also calculate the **extra** risk in smokers over and above the risk in non-smokers (49 – 7 = 42 deaths per 100 000 smokers per year). We are saying that there is a rate of lung cancer deaths (7 per 100 000 people) which is due to causes other than smoking, such as genes or exposure to environmental radon gas. It is there in the non-smokers and even if the smokers did not smoke they would still experience this mortality risk.

So we partition the total risk of dying of lung cancer if you are a smoker (49 per 100 000 per year) into two parts:

- 7 deaths per 100 000 smokers per year which are unconnected to smoking because this is the risk in non-smokers as well.
- 42 deaths per 100 000 smokers per year which represents the extra risk of dying from lung cancer because of smoking. This is called the **excess** or **attributable risk**.

Why bother? Why not stick to risk ratios, which are much simpler to grasp. Here is one reason.

- As a smoker, you are 1.4 times more likely to die of heart disease than a non-smoker.

Smokers have an added risk of coronary heart disease, but it seems to be a much weaker link than that between smoking and lung cancer. However, coronary heart disease is much more common than lung cancer and the death rate from it is much higher than for lung cancer. So the patient's question '1.4 times more likely than what?' becomes interesting.

Mortality rate from coronary heart disease:

- 1000 deaths per 100 000 smokers per year;
- 700 deaths per 100 000 non-smokers per year.

The excess risk of dying from coronary heart disease in smokers which can be attributed to smoking itself is thus an extra 300 deaths per 100 000 smokers per year: considerably more deaths than can be attributed to the link between smoking and lung cancer (42 per 100 000 smokers per year). Smoking has a greater impact on coronary heart disease mortality because the latter is so much more common than lung cancer.

The step from relative measures of association to absolute measures of risk is an important one for the critical reader, because it is about making the results of studies and trials relevant to the individual patient. It is an important part of the *reflective* aspect of critical appraisal of published material.

> The West of Scotland trial of cholesterol reduction in healthy middle-aged men showed an overall benefit expressed as a 30% reduction in mortality in men on active drug therapy (West of Scotland Coronary Prevention Group, 1996). However, if we take a specific group, such as smokers, the results show that smokers on active cholesterol-lowering treatment still had a higher mortality than non-smokers in the control group taking placebo treatment. Paradoxically the absolute risk reduction is still more marked in those with the higher coronary risk, such as smokers, because their risk is higher to begin with.
>
> The authors of the study went one step further and calculated the reduction in actual risk: 6% in those initially at high risk of a coronary event and 1.5% in those at low risk. Expressed in another way, 17 high-risk patients would need to be treated to prevent one cardiovascular event compared with 66 low-risk patients needing to be treated to prevent one event.

The process is part of teasing out the **generalizability** of study results, helping to develop a picture of the **external validity** of the study and identifying the particular individuals to whom the results of a study might be applied with benefit in actual practice.

Oral contraceptives appear to carry an overall risk of deep venous thrombosis, but what is the actual risk? Are some groups of women at higher risk than others? How does the risk compare to the risks of DVT in pregnancy? Table 5.1 summarizes some published figures which build up this picture, adapted from Guillebaud (1995).

Of course, absolute risks and benefits do not give a simple prescription of right and wrong actions. It is less a case of a single critical question 'Is this study valid for my patients or not?' than a case of 'If I believe this result, let me work out in which groups of patients it might be most important or effective or useful – and put

Table 5.1 Risk of venous thromboembolism

	Relative risk	*Actual risk per 100 000 women per year*
Healthy non-pregnant women, not taking hormones	1*	5
Women in the year of a pregnancy	12	60
Women taking 2nd generation oral contraceptives	3	15
Women taking 3rd generation oral contraceptives	6	30

*Taken as the baseline risk.

a figure on that'. Risk is a difficult area for explaining to patients and is addressed further in Chapter 9.

TEST YOURSELF: STATISTICS

SUMMARY STATISTICS: MARGARINE EATING AND BLOOD FAT

In a study to establish the effects of margarine on lipid levels in the blood (Chisholm, 1996), the results started as follows: '49 subjects (35 women, 14 men), mean age 46.8 (SD 11.6) years, completed the 21-week protocol. Initial mean body mass index was 26.4 (3.8) kg/m^2'.

Questions

1 How else could you summarize the gender distribution of the sample?
2 What does (SD 11.6) tell you about the sample?
3 What does the use of the mean as the summary statistic tell you about the distribution of age and body mass index in this sample? What additional statistic might help you to judge this?

Suggested answers

1 71% of the sample were women.
2 68% of this sample were aged between 35 and 58 years *or* 95% of this sample were aged between 23 and 70 years.
3 It assumes that the ages and body mass indices follow a normal distribution. Age, weight and height do have a normal distribution in the general population. However, this sample is not very big and we might want convincing that the distributions do approximate to the normal bell-shaped curve. If the medians were provided as well and if they coincide with the means, this would increase our confidence that the data are normally distributed. Alternatively, scatterplots of the individual readings would help the reader to assess the distribution visually.

STATISTICAL TESTING AND ESTIMATING

Example I: treatment of low back pain

Table 5.2 shows the changes in a disability score in patients with low back pain. They were participants in a randomized trial which allocated them to receive hospital-based physiotherapy or treatment by a chiropractor (Meade, 1990). They were followed up for 2 years.

Questions: example I

1 What does $P<0.05$ mean?
2 What does $P<0.01$ mean?
3 Put into words the 95% confidence interval for the mean difference at 6 months. How does it relate to the P value?
4 Why does the 95% confidence interval for the mean difference at 12 months not have an asterisk?
5 What problem might be created by the dropout rate during the study, shown by the declining numbers of patients used in the analysis at each successive follow-up point?
6 What statistical test might have been used to calculate the P values for the difference in the mean disability changes?
7 What further information would you like in order to judge whether this is an important result for general practice or not?

Table 5.2 Changes in disability scores from baseline: mean difference between physiotherapy and chiropractic groups

	6 months	*12 months*	*24 months*
Mean difference in changes in disability score	3.3*	2.1	7.2**
95% confidence interval	(0.5 to 6.1)	(−1.1 to +5.3)	(1.9 to 12.5)
Numbers in physiotherapy group	282	207	90
Numbers in chiropractic group	325	247	104

* $P<0.05$
** $P<0.01$
Source: Meade (1990)

Suggested answers: example I

1 This is the traditional cut-off point which defines 'statistical significance'. Suppose the observed differences in disability change had happened because of chance differences in the two groups after randomization, rather than to a true difference in the effects of the two interventions. If the 'truth' in this example were 'no difference between the two groups' (the null hypothesis), the result actually observed would have arisen by chance on fewer than 1 occasion in 20 such random experiments ($P = 0.05 = 5$ in $100 = 1$ in 20). This is regarded as 'unlikely' and so the interpretation is that this is a 'real' rather than a random difference. Whether the result is then attributed to the interventions will depend on an analysis of possible biases in the study.

2 This indicates a result even less likely to have arisen by chance ($P = 0.01 = 1$ in 100). If there were 'truly' no difference between the groups, this result would have arisen by chance on fewer than 1 in 100 occasions involving similarly sized and designed randomized experiments.

3 The 95% confidence interval gives an estimate of the chance variation we might expect in the result if the experiment was

repeated many times. It provides a range within which we can be 95% confident that the 'real' mean difference between the treatments might lie. At 6 months the interval does not include zero. So the 'no difference' hypothesis is unlikely: equivalent to a *P* value of <0.05 and a rejection of the null hypothesis.

4 At 12 months the 95% confidence interval does include zero. If 'no difference' were true, this result would have arisen by chance more frequently than 1 in 20 occasions – so the *P* value is >0.05 and the observed difference is not statistically significant.

5 All the arguments above about 'truth' and 'chance' depend entirely on the assumption that the study is unbiased and that any differences observed are due to chance differences following randomization or real differences attributable to the interventions. If dropout has occurred for different reasons in the two groups, then the result might represent bias rather than truth or chance variation. Suppose that chiropractic patients dropped out of follow-up if they did not get better, whereas physiotherapy patients dropped out if they improved. This would make the two follow-up groups appear different even if chiropractic therapy and physiotherapy had identical effects on low back disability.

6 A comparison of means when standard deviations are quoted can be assumed to be based on the normal distribution, and *t* tests are one approach to the analysis of such data.

7 This question is not about the mechanism of statistical analysis but about *reflecting* on the possible importance of the results to your practice.

- How were the patients selected for the trial prior to randomization? Could the results apply to low back pain patients in general or does the study population represent a highly select minority?
- What does the difference in disability score mean – does it have clinical relevance, would it be important to the individual patient?
- Are there subgroups in which the differences were clear-cut and others in which there was no difference?
- What were the actual interventions used in the study and how could they be introduced, at what cost and for how long, in general practice?

Example II: the psychological effect of screening

This question is taken from the paper by Stoate, laid out in Chapter 2 (Stoate, 1989).

The general health questionnaire (GHQ) is a well validated self-completion instrument, which identifies individuals with possible clinical depression and anxiety. The results of a GHQ survey were compared at baseline and 3 months later within a group (the 'study' group) of primary care patients who attended at baseline for cardiovascular screening and were found to be healthy. The change in the study group was compared with GHQ scores obtained at parallel points in time from a group of randomly chosen controls.

Table 5.3 Percentage of respondents with GHQ score >5 (95% confidence intervals in brackets)

	Baseline GHQ	*3-month GHQ*	
Screened group ($n = 189$)	21.7 (15.2 to 26.8)	35.4 (28.2 to 41.8)	$\chi^2 = 8.1$ $P<0.05$
Control group ($n = 155$)	34.1 (26.6 to 41.4)	25.8 (18.0 to 32.0)	$\chi^2 = 2.2$ not significant

Questions: example II

1 What does 'not significant' mean?
2 Why has a chi-square test been used?
3 Assuming that GHQ scores of more than 5 indicate that patients are more likely to be clinically depressed, how would you interpret the results?
4 Is the comparison of the two groups reasonable?

Suggested answers: example II

1 Not significant means not significant **statistically**. It is based on the 'P' or probability value, which indicates the likelihood that an observed result has arisen by chance. If there was no difference between the groups and the observed result could have arisen by

chance on more than 1 out of 20 occasions with a similar size and design of trial, the observed difference is said to be non-significant and the null hypothesis of 'no difference between the groups' is accepted.

2 The GHQ score has been categorized so that the study subjects are in two groups: those with a score above 5 and those with a score of 5 or below. The proportions in the two groups have been compared between baseline and 3 months to see if they have changed. The chi-square test can be used for such a comparison of frequencies.

3 The results displayed suggest that, 3 months after cardiovascular screening in primary care, 14% of patients who had no abnormality on screening are likely to become depressed. Since a control group did not show a similar increase in the proportion with depression, one explanation is that the screening procedure itself might be responsible for precipitating psychological upset.

4 The problem with the comparison displayed is that the study group and control group are not the same on the first occasion: the proportion of patients who were depressed at baseline was higher in the control group. This may invalidate the between-group comparison of changes in scores from baseline to follow-up. Like is not being compared with like.

ESTIMATING EFFECTS

Example I: ozone levels and wheezing in children

In a study of children attending casualty departments with acute wheezy episodes (Buchdahl, 1996), the risk ratio was 3.1 for the comparison between attendance on days when the ozone concentration was lower than the annual average and attendance on days with an ozone concentration equal to the average over 1 year.

Question: example I

What does the risk ratio mean?

Suggested answer: example I

The risk ratio is a measure of association. It would appear from this brief extract that the study was looking for an association between ozone concentration and acute wheeze. A comparison has been made between the risk of patients attending Casualty with wheeze on days when ozone concentrations are low and the risk of attending on days when ozone concentrations are close to the annual average. This comparison has been summarized by dividing one risk by another: the ratio obtained gives a summary of the association (a three times higher risk that wheezy attenders will attend on low ozone days compared with average days).

Example II: physical activity and heart disease

Table 5.4 shows the mortality from coronary heart disease in men, according to physical activity. These figures are taken from a prospective cohort study (Paffenbarger, 1975) of men from the same industry, who have different types of job. These figures have been adjusted to remove any effect of different ages of the men in the three different activity categories.

Table 5.4

Physical activity level	*Relative risk of dying from CHD*
Heavy	1.0
Moderate	3.5
Light	2.8

Questions: example II

1 What does relative risk mean?
2 What is a prospective study?
3 Why was adjusting for age important?
4 How would you interpret the study?

Suggested answers: example II

1 The probability of developing coronary disease among men who have jobs involving moderate physical activity is 3.5 times that

among men with jobs involving heavy physical activity. The relative risk of coronary disease is then said to be 3.5 for moderate compared with heavy occupational activity in men.

2 A prospective study is 'forward-looking'. Information is first gathered about possible causes or influences on the onset or the outcome of the problem under investigation. The persons being studied are then followed up over time to determine the start of the outcome of that problem. It tries to observe and measure 'cause' before 'effect'.

3 Coronary disease in men becomes more common with age. Levels of physical activity and types of job involving heavy activity are likely to change with age. Any study which attempts to link physical activity to coronary disease must ensure that it is not simply studying the effect of age on both.

4 From the data provided, it would seem that coronary mortality is less common in men who have jobs involving heavy levels of physical activity. One interpretation is that physical activity protects against coronary disease; however it may be that it protects against death from coronary disease rather than against the disease itself.

There is no obvious trend of increasing risk with decreasing activity. We would need to know whether it is something about men who undertake heavy activity specifically which is protecting them before interpreting the results as meaning exercise is good for the heart.

Example III: vitamin supplementation and prevention of neural tube defects

For the next two questions, we will look again at some data from Chapter 4, specifically the 'Test yourself' section concerning vitamin supplementation and the prevention of neural tube defects (p. 88)

Questions: example III

1 First, in question 3 (p.88), the prospective observational study had a data table as follows:

Table 5.5 Number of pregnancies by outcome and vitamin supplementation

| | Vitamin supplementation | |
	Yes	No
Neural tube defects	1	13
No neural tube defects	178	260

a What is the risk of a child having a neural tube defect when mothers choose to take vitamins?
b What is the risk for children whose mothers do not take regular vitamins?
c What is the risk ratio for the association between mothers *not* taking regular vitamins and their children having a neural tube defect?
d Put the risk ratio into words.

2 Turning now to the randomized controlled trial (question 4, p.88).

Table 5.6 Numbers of pregnancies by outcome and vitamin supplementation

| | Intervention | |
	Vitamin	Placebo
Neural tube defects	6	21
No neural tube defects	593	602

a What is the risk ratio based on the trial?
b Why is this ratio different to the risk ratio derived from the observational study above?
c What are the actual reductions in risk which might be achieved by vitamin supplementation around conception in women with a prior history of a child with a neural tube defect? Derive two separate answers from the two studies (observational and RCT).

Suggested answers: example III

1 a The absolute risk of a child having an NTD among mothers
   taking vitamins in the observational study was 1/179, i.e. 5.6
   per 1000 births.
  b The absolute risk for mothers not taking vitamins in that
   study was 13/273, i.e. 47.6 per 1000 births.
  c The risk ratio is thus 47.6 divided by 5.6, i.e. 8.5.
  d Put into words, this means that the risk of having a child
   with a neural tube defect (NTD) among mothers who have a
   previous history of an NTD-affected pregnancy is 8.5 times
   higher in women who could not recall taking vitamin supplements at the time of conception compared with those who
   recalled taking supplements.
2 a In the randomized controlled trial a similar calculation shows
   the risks to be 10.0 per 1000 births in women allocated to
   take vitamins compared with 33.7 per 1000 births in women
   taking placebo tablets. The risk ratio is thus 33.7 divided by
   10.0, i.e. 3.4.
  b In the intervention trial, the risks in the two groups are closer
   together than in the observational study: the risk in vitamin
   takers is higher than in the corresponding group in the
   observational study, whereas the risk in the non-vitamin
   takers is lower.
   The first explanation is that randomization may have
   removed potential confounders. Women who choose to take
   vitamins may differ in many ways from women who do not
   take vitamins: and some of those ways may be linked to the
   likelihood of an NTD pregnancy. Other parts of their diet,
   smoking, alcohol, are all possible examples. In the trial the
   chance of getting active or placebo vitamin was decided
   randomly, so all these other factors should have been distributed roughly evenly between the two groups. If this is
   true, then the risk ratio in the trial is a **more valid estimate**
   of the association between vitamin taking and NTD
   prevention.
   There is another approach however. This says that women
   who agree to take part in trials are themselves unusual, not
   representative of all women with previous NTD-affected
   pregnancies. Although the comparison between the placebo
   and active groups in the trial still gives a 'pure' answer to the

question of whether vitamins actually reduce NTD risk or not, the absolute risks measured may not represent the real world. So it may be the risks from the observational study which give a closer answer to the question: 'What are the likely outcomes if women with a previous history are advised to take vitamins at the time of conception?'.

c The risk reduction attributable to vitamin supplementation, based on the observational data would be

$$47.6 - 5.6 = 42.0 \text{ fewer events per 1000 births}$$

among women with a previous history.

From the intervention trial the estimated reduction would be

$$33.7 - 10.0 = 23.7 \text{ fewer events per 1000 births}$$

among women with a previous history.

REFERENCES

Buchdahl, R., Parker, A., Stebbings, T., and Babiker, A. (1996) Association between air pollution and acute childhood wheezy episodes: prospective observational study. *British Medical Journal*, **312**, 661–5.

Campbell, M.J., and Machin, D. (1993) *Medical statistics. A commonsense approach*. Chichester: John Wiley and Sons.

Chisholm, A., Mann, J., Sutherland, W., Duncan, A., Skeaff, M., and Frampton, C. (1996). Effect on lipoprotein profile of replacing butter with margarine in a low fat diet: crossover study with hypercholesterolaemic subjects. *British Medical Journal*, **312**, 931–4.

Coggon, D. (1995) *Statistics in Clinical Practice*. BMJ Publishing Group.

Doll, R., and Peto, R. (1976) Mortality in relation to smoking: 20 years' observations on male British doctors. *British Medical Journal*, **(ii)**, 1525–36.

Guillebaud, J. (1995) Advising women on which pill to take. *British Medical Journal*, **311**, 1111–2.

Meade, T.W., Dyer, S., Browne, W., Townsend, J., and Frank, A.O. (1990) Low back pain of mechanical origin: randomised comparison of chiropractic and hospital outpatient treatment. *British Medical Journal*, **300**, 1431–7.

Paffenbarger, R.S. and Hale, W.E. (1975) Work activity and coronary heart mortality. *New England Journal of Medicine*, **292**, 545–50.

Stoate, H.G. (1989) Can health screening damage your health? *Journal of the Royal College of General Practitioners*, **39**, 193–5.

West of Scotland Coronary Prevention Group, (1996) West of Scotland Coronary Prevention Study: Identification of high-risk groups and comparison with other cardiovascular intervention trials. *Lancet*, **348**, 1339–42.

6

Reflecting on a study: implications for practice

The first response of the critical reader to a lot of published research is 'so what?'. The implications of a study result need to be considered as thoughtfully as the design and methods. The stakes are high: an error in applying a research finding may have consequences for the health of patients and the resources of the practice.

Drawing implications

If we were to admit a prejudice, it is that the heart of critical appraisal lies here. Not in the obsessive analysis of the methods and design – important as these are – but in the universally accessible skills of logical, experience-based **critical reflection** on what the study implies for your own practice.

Some of the limitations of a study should have been pointed out by the authors in their discussion, but by using a systematic approach, you can often spot other important points which the authors have ignored. The broad approach described in this chapter should help you to generate more than enough ideas about the extent to which implications can be drawn from a published paper. Once you start practising such an approach, you will find that the 'critical points' about implications seem easier to spot. This is the next step after that first 'so what?'.

A framework

It helps to have a framework for thinking through the different implications of a study. A helpful starting point is to divide **implications** into two broad components: generalizability and consequences.

Jargon corner

Two components of implications

1 **Generalizability**: the extent to which a result might apply in the world outside the study
2 **Consequences**: given that it might be possible to generalize the result of the study to other situations, what would be the practical consequences of this?

When the term 'implications' is used, most people think first about the obvious practical **consequences** for primary care and miss out the first and more critical component which is a consideration of **generalizability**. For this reason we will start by considering the process of making such generalizations.

GENERALIZATION OF STUDY RESULTS

This involves much more than the simple statement 'these results could be replicated in situations similar to those described in the study'. Replication of a study may be an important issue, but even if an identical study produced identical results, there would still be valid questions to ask about how the context of the study relates to other situations, particularly to the rough and tumble of real primary care.

The Geoffrey Rose rule

As you start to consider whether a study can be generalized, be clear about the *objective* of the study. The late Geoffrey Rose, who was

Professor of Epidemiology at The London School of Hygiene and Tropical Medicine and a great supporter of primary care research, would remind students when they were in full critical flow that they should not take a study to task for something which it did not set out to investigate. We refer to this as the Geoffrey Rose rule: focus critical reading on features of direct relevance to the objectives the study has set itself.

Summary box

The Geoffrey Rose rule

- Focus on study features relevant to the **objective** of the study.
- Don't ask something of the study which it did not set out to do

---

The broad idea is illustrated in Figure 6.1. The next sections then detail the framework for dividing the methods and results of a study into a number of categories to ask, 'Can we reasonably generalize from this particular study to primary care in general?'.

The study setting

The first obvious question is whether the research has been carried out in primary care. If it has, consider what sort of practice populations were represented by the practice or practices studied. Care is needed to relate any 'unrepresentativeness' to the purpose of the study.

Example: diabetes in primary care

A study to estimate the prevalence of diabetes in a practice population is planned. The study practice might differ in crucial ways – ethnicity, age structure – from other practices, so the prevalence figure could only be applied cautiously to other practices even if the study itself was excellent.

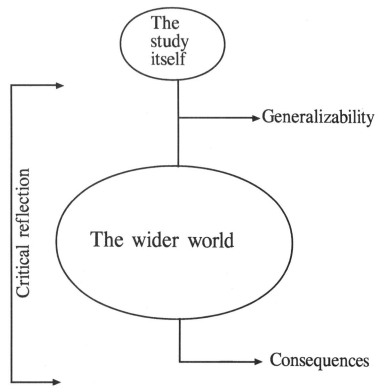

Figure 6.1 The place of critical reflection.

Consider, by contrast, the question: 'What is the association between diabetic complications and poor diabetic control in a general practice population?'. This is more generalizable. The answer can be applied independently of the actual frequency of diabetes in a practice.

A study from outside primary care will influence the extent to which implications may be drawn. For example, suppose a study concluded that an EEG and brain scan are very helpful investigations in patients presenting with dizziness. You might suspect that this study had not taken place in general practice or even in a district general hospital. Most likely it would have been based on patients seen in a specialist neurology referral centre. General practitioners would be rightly wary of extrapolating such a result to patients who are consulting for the first time in their surgeries because of dizziness. A recent study of dizziness in the general population supports such caution (Colledge, 1996).

However, the results of studies which have not been done in general practice are often applicable or relevant to primary care. For example, suppose a trial of two types of inhaler in an outpatient chest clinic demonstrates a clear superiority of one inhaler over the other. This might be reasonably generalized to a similar group of patients in primary care (e.g. patients with asthma of comparable severity). Studying this in an outpatients' setting might be the most efficient way to identify a sufficiently large number of patients. The context is not crucial if the question is about **efficacy** (does one inhaler work better?).

Equally we cannot assume that a study carried out in general practice will necessarily provide results of general relevance.

> The trial of once daily amoxycillin versus usual dose penicillin for pharyngitis, described in detail earlier (Shvartzman, 1993), suggested amoxycillin might be better at eradicating strepto-cocci from the throat. Whether or not such a result was relevant to your practice would depend on knowing about many other aspects of the study (patient selection, diagnosis of pharyngitis, whether eradicating streptococci is an important issue in treating sore throat, costs and side-effects of the two regimes) rather than the single fact that it was based in general practice.

The subjects studied

Even when the setting is primary care, generalization may be constrained by case definition.

> A study of hypertension and stroke is published. Subjects were identified as hypertensive from a review of computerized repeat prescriptions. This may be a valid and unbiased study of such patients, but we cannot necessarily generalize this to all hypertensives in a practice population (who may also include the undiscovered, the untreated, those managed without drugs or those treated with drugs but not on the computerized repeat prescription system).

How we generalize and the implications we draw will depend on the question being asked.

> In the example above, suppose the question was: 'Is the risk of stroke in patients who receive repeat prescriptions for anti-hypertensive drugs related to the quality of blood pressure monitoring?'. The result could be generalized to all hypertensives on repeat prescriptions.
>
> Take a different question: 'What is the impact on stroke incidence of treating hypertension in general practice?'. Here we must be more cautious about drawing conclusions from a study group defined by regular drug therapy. Such a group will not include all hypertensives in a practice (those on non-pharmacological treatment, for example, will be excluded). Hypertensive patients who do not receive repeat prescriptions are an important part of the equation when a general statement about treating hypertension in general practice is made.

Classic examples where generalizations have been made and then proven to be mistaken are to be found in the field of drug trials. New non-steroidal anti-inflammatory drugs, for example, may conveniently be tested in young adults with musculoskeletal problems, and be shown to be effective with no untoward effects. If these results are then generalized to common musculoskeletal problems in primary care, one thing is certain, the bulk of recipients will be patients from a completely different age group to those in the trials, namely the elderly.

> This is what happened with 'Opren', a drug which appeared to offer unusual efficacy in the treatment of osteoarthritis. It brought the promise of beneficial effects on the disease process itself as well as on the symptoms of pain and stiffness. Introduced with a fanfare, it was withdrawn after a number of reports of severe reactions among elderly patients taking the drug, including some deaths. Most general practice patients with painful osteoarthritis are over 60; results of the pre-launch trials were extrapolated to this age group by the very act of advertising the drug as an important treatment for osteoarthritis in primary care. The side-effects, which subsequently emerged as exclusively affecting the elderly and which led to the

withdrawal of the drug, were a visible demonstration of faulty generalization which transferred the results in one population (the young) to a population crucially different in its response to the drug (the elderly).

The intervention

An intervention might have been introduced specifically as part of the study – as in a trial for instance – or observed as part of usual care or practice. To what extent can it be generalized?

Screening for occult blood in faeces has been claimed to be a sensitive method of identifying lower gut cancer. However, the context of that 'sensitivity' must be examined carefully: Would the process be acceptable in primary care patients? Would sufficient people take it up and be prepared to repeat it to make it worthwhile? Did the result depend on a dedicated research team of doctors and nurses which simply would not be available in 'routine' primary care? Was participation in the study itself likely to have improved the outcome?

The answers depend on the tricky process of judging how the circumstances and the techniques of a particular study might work out in actual practice.

End-points

Studies are confined to the end-points they choose to investigate.

Studies of breast cancer screening are beginning to point to a general reduction in mortality. Because a screening programme reduces mortality, it does not follow that it is successful from other points of view – such as relief of symptoms or improved quality of life or satisfaction with screening and with the subsequent treatment.

It is appropriate, in considering the implications of a study, to ask whether end-points other than those reported might be relevant and important.

Studies of drugs for painful conditions are often short-term. Although relief of immediate symptoms is important, the major burden on primary care often comes from those patients in whom pain becomes chronic. Generalizing from short-term efficacy to long-term benefit may be flawed.

The actual result

Look at the actual size of a result and calculate the likely practical or clinical effect of a finding. This may be different to the result emphasized by the authors, who may have highlighted a statistical test of significance for example.

The effect of salt restriction in reducing blood pressure in the study described in the introductory chapter was statistically significant (MacGregor, 1989). This was important as a contribution to the debate about whether national nutritional policy should include restriction of salt intake. Yet the result could not easily be extrapolated to everyday clinical practice because the size of the blood pressure fall achieved was small relative to the extent of the restriction needed to treat the individual patient.

Summary box: generalizability

Setting: Is it applicable to primary care patients?

Subjects: Are they representative of unselected patients?

Intervention: Would it be acceptable and replicable outside the study setting?

End-points: Are they relevant to actual practice?

Result: How big an effect has been observed in the study and how important is it clinically?

A SPECIAL PROBLEM FOR GENERALIZATION: THE RANDOMIZED CONTROLLED TRIAL

A favourite type of study for journals to publish is the randomized controlled trial. Such trials are often elegant in design and they most closely resemble a scientific experiment. The influence of confounding variables which might affect the result is removed by the process of random allocation to an intervention group and a control group.

Paradoxically, despite the strong design, the major problem posed by a controlled trial is often that of generalizability. Rigorous selection of suitable subjects often occurs and the exclusion of many subjects from entry into a trial limits its applicability. The more selective a trial becomes, the harder it becomes to generalize the results.

Reflection stop

RCTs and generalizability

1 Randomized controlled trials are scientifically elegant.
2 It may not be easy to generalize from the restricted study population of a randomized controlled trial to wider groups of patients.

In considering how far generalizations can be made from a trial, the aim of the trial is crucial. A useful distinction to make is whether the study is attempting to be 'explanatory' or 'pragmatic' in purpose and design. (This links closely with the section in Chapter 4 about 'Intention to treat'.)

An example will help to illustrate these two terms. You want to know whether antibiotics are helpful in the treatment of sore throat in primary care.

The trial of amoxycillin and penicillin V in the treatment of pharyngitis in primary care suggested that once-daily amoxycillin was more efficacious than four times daily penicillin V in eradicating streptococci from the throat.

If the bacteriological results seem trustworthy and the likeliest explanation of the eradication of streptococci was the efficacy of amoxycillin, then you have a piece of evidence from an **explanatory** trial. But this has not answered the question: Are antibiotics useful in practice?

> You read the study again and note a number of problems: most of the patients in the trial did not have streptococci in their throats at the end of a 10-day period, regardless of the drug they were taking, and there seemed to be no difference between the groups with respect to symptom improvement.

This explanatory trial had a specific focus: was there any difference between the two drug regimes with respect to one outcome: eradication of streptococci. The result could be applied to a particular patient group (patients with sore throat who had a positive throat swab for streptococcus and received penicillin in one form or other).

You, however, want to find out whether treating sore throat with antibiotics is effective at improving the clinical problem (sore throat), and you know that improvement in real life might be influenced by patients' expectations, by compliance with taking the drugs, and by natural resolution of the condition, as much as any specifically anti-bacterial effect of the drugs. You turn to a different sort of trial.

> Little *et al.* (1997) described an 'open' randomized trial. This is a trial which is not placebo controlled, and not double-blinded. The study setting was in 11 general practices, and patients with sore throat were randomized to three groups: to receive a prescription for a 10-day course of antibiotics, to receive a prescription to start antibiotics only if symptoms were not better within 3 days, and to receive no prescription.

No throat swabs, no bacteriological outcomes, no placebo group, no blinding: heretical stuff. Not everyone with a sore throat was recruited, so the population may not have been entirely representative of all sore throats in general practice. However, the point of the study was to find out overall how patients fared on these three practical strategies, attempting in particular to mimic the influences on outcome which might happen in actual practice (patient knowledge, expectations, satisfaction and so on).

The proportion of patients better by the third day was no different between the three groups.

This does not rule out the possibility that, in those who were taking the antibiotic, streptococci were being eradicated more quickly. Nor does it allow us to disentangle the reasons for recovery. What it loses in precise explanation, it gains in generalizability to the general practice situation. Overall, the choice to prescribe a 10-day course of antibiotics does not improve your patients' chances of getting better from their sore throat. A practical answer from a pragmatic trial.

However, you are not left with an answer to the very specific question posed by the explanatory trial: How useful are antibiotics at eradicating streptococci? You would need to know whether this outcome was important (e.g. perhaps complications in a small group of patients are reduced, but current evidence suggests it does not provide a good rationale for treating sore throats with antibiotics). The usefulness of a trial relates to its aim and its principal outcome, as well as to the population it has studied.

The important point to note is that if you wish to generalize a result to general practice, a trial based on a 'pragmatic' question is likely to be better. If you look at an explanatory trial which explores factors which may be of scientific interest but which does not address the question of 'How might this work in practice', implications may be more difficult to draw.

CONSEQUENCES OF STUDY RESULTS

The second component of implications relates to consequences. It is important to take a broad view of the practical consequences of applying the findings of a study. Here we are asking:

'Whatever my reservations about the extent to which these results can be generalized, what would actually happen if they were applied in my practice or in other practices?'

Thinking about the full range of consequences is part of the process of **critical reflection** on the implications of a study in which only the narrower consequences have been explicitly drawn out or discussed by the authors.

When considering consequences, it is important to think broadly and often 'brain storming' is a useful strategy. If you have difficulty thinking of specific consequences of a study and your 'brain storming' dries up, it may help to have a reminder of some of the important areas to consider. One such list is shown below.

Reflection stop

Consequences
How might the following be affected by putting the study result into practice?

● The patients and their families.
● The doctors and the practice partnership.
● The primary health care team.
● Practice issues: prescribing, costs, standard setting, audit.
● Need for protocols.
● Broad implications for society and the local community.
● Ethical issues.

Summary box: critical reflection and implications

It is helpful to divide implications into two components:

1 **Generalizability**: the extent to which results might apply outside the study
2 **Consequences**: given that the results of the study can be generalized (with or without reservations), what would be the practical consequences of applying them?

Checklist for generalizations

Setting   comparable to general practice?

Subjects   representative of which patients?

Intervention acceptable? replicable outside study?

End-points are other end-points relevant?

Result how large an effect and how important clinically?

Checklist for consequences

T Time and training (GP, the team, the patient)
R Resources (workload and money)
A Audit (includes standard setting, protocols, follow-up)
P People (patient, doctor, practice)
S Safety and society (includes ethical issues)

TEST YOURSELF: DRAWING IMPLICATIONS

We will now consider the implications for practice of three different papers. The discussion aims to illustrate the process of thinking critically about implications and the boxes highlight some of the main points. This is about critical reflection: the application of critical reading or research papers to real life.

Try each example before comparing your thoughts with ours.

THE CASE FOR NICOTINE PATCHES

Question

What are the implications for general practice? Try answering the question before you read the box and text below. Give yourself 15 minutes to answer the question.

Consider a follow-up report of a randomized controlled trial in primary care (ICRF General Practice Research Group, 1994). This paper reported the 12-month follow-up results of a trial in primary care of nicotine versus placebo patches as an aid to smoking cessation in subjects smoking 15 or more cigarettes daily. The previously reported difference in cessation rates 3 months after intervention (19% in nicotine group versus 12% in placebo group) was shown to persist at 1 year, although some early abstainers in both groups had resumed the habit by 12 months (continuing abstinence at 1 year 11% in nicotine group versus 8% in placebo group). The difference between active and placebo treatment was smaller at 1 year than it had been at 3 months.

We will assume that you as the reader are happy with the conduct of the study: that the groups were similar in all respects except the nature of the substance in the patches, that the measurements of smoking cessation were valid, and that the trial was large enough. In other words the trial appeared free of bias and the result precise.

Let us now consider the two components of critical reflection on the implications of a study: generalization and consequences.

Generalization

Study setting

This study was carried out in general practice, with general practice patients, which means that the results are potentially relevant to primary care as a whole. However, it might help to know more of the general characteristics of the practices involved. This, of course, should not in theory affect the result of a randomized comparison of patients within the practices (some getting nicotine, some not), but it might be relevant to the baseline rate of smoking cessation. If these were unusually enthusiastic practices in areas where the clientele are likely to place a generally high priority on preventive health, then the likelihood of finding smokers motivated to stop may be high, and the extra effect imparted by a nicotine patch might appear clinically worthwhile pursuing. Turn to practices with less motivation and higher fallout rates and the additional benefit of a nicotine patch effect might be so small as to be of questionable value.

The study population

A problem with randomized controlled trials is that they necessarily consist of people who are prepared to give consent to take part and in whom the investigators are happy to encourage that participation. The more exclusions that are made prior to randomization, the more precisely the specific research question may be answered (so, for example, having a group of smokers motivated to take part in a trial may help to ensure good follow-up attendance and persistence with the intervention). The down side is that the results become less easy to generalize to all patients who might benefit. If most smokers in your practice are smoking less than 15 cigarettes per day, and are poorly motivated to stop, then as an intervention to reduce smoking in your practice, the nicotine patch may be a poor choice.

However, too much agonizing of this sort will neutralize the ability of a trial to offer any help to practitioners at all. It is the problem of getting some good scientific evidence on a basic question (the explanatory trial) versus the need to know whether the intervention would be useful in practice (the pragmatic trial). Here it can be rephrased as 'now that I know nicotine patches can have a beneficial effect of some sort, how much can I reasonably extrapolate beyond the actual situation described in the trial?'. Carefully judged generalization is both reasonable and necessary. What proportion of subjects in a practice might be heavy smokers?; what proportion of all smokers does this represent?; how many people were asked to take part in this trial and what proportion agreed? Knowing the answers to such questions would help to judge the extent to which this study population can be generalized.

The study process

In this study the intervention involved initial doctor advice, follow-up support and outcome measurement by research nurses. This implies quite hefty resources. Some of this is necessitated by the trial itself, but questions follow about their generalizability. How much might these trial processes have contributed, for example, to the important benefit in the placebo group? Could such influences be replicated in everyday practice? What about the costs, the personnel, the digression from other work in the practice? Of course it can be argued that the main effect was a therapeutic nicotine effect, but, as the authors themselves point out, this effect was observed in the context of doctor and nurse support for motivated subjects, and they doubt whether a nicotine effect would be observed in the absence of such a background.

So results cannot necessarily be generalized (nicotine does good) without the attendant baggage. This may carry cost and resource implications as well as doubts as to whether the trial intervention could be applied in reality.

End-points

A good effect at 3 months is a helpful start in assessing the potential of nicotine patches, but is rather remote from the pragmatics of practice where short-term cessation cannot be assumed to be an improvement on refusing to give up in the first place. If short-term cessation is a marker for longer-term abstinence, then the results would have more important implications. The follow-up to 1 year offers some evidence for such a continuing effect, but also highlights a narrowing of the difference between active and placebo groups. The real long-term value of the nicotine must be open to question, whilst the 1-year results begin to suggest that the support structure (doctors, nurses) is relatively more important than the drug.

However, the Geoffrey Rose rule should be recalled. This study did not set out to answer the question of the value of putting dedicated nurses into a smoking reduction programme in general practice. That particular intervention was not randomized, it was given to everyone. Perhaps doctor advice alone would be as effective as nurse support – you would need evidence from other studies to judge that. The only **direct** implication is that, if you did introduce a programme of advice with doctor and nurse participation, then adding a patch of nicotine would confer a small but definite additional benefit.

The actual result

Judging the result itself must include a review of the actual figures presented, not simply the statistical significance of a result, but rather the implications of the numbers presented. Here the argument would run that if you put everyone onto nicotine patches, 3% would still be there abstaining 1 year later because of the nicotine rather than any other aspect of your programme (3% being the difference between the proportion of abstainers in the nicotine and placebo groups).

Now that may be expensive on money, resources and time, and it still does not mean that nicotine would produce a similar result without the other programme interventions, but it does give a flavour of what could actually be achieved.

Put in more realistic terms with respect to numbers, if you identified 100 such patients in your practice, gave them all the programme, 11 would have been abstaining from cigarettes a year later if nicotine patches were used, and 8 would have stopped if patches had not been used. (Even this is not strictly true for it ignores the effect of the placebo patch – without any patch at all the number might be lower than 8.)

Consequences

Whether such an effort is worthwhile in practice is part of a broader view, involving for example:

● Costs
● Staffing resources and training in health promotion.
● The need for a continuing programme for it to be effective in the long term and the need to audit the interventions given.
● The balance between helping individuals who would respond to the patch, and the much lower pay-off for your whole community of smoking patients, most of whom would not benefit. Long-term effects include: some good (maybe getting them started on the road to cessation has a general knock-on effect; having a smoking cessation programme may have a wider influence on smoking habits within the practice; nurses and doctors may quickly get geared to it being part of regular anticipatory care); some bad (gradual decline in the impact of the patch over time might mean the whole thing just is not worthwhile in the long run; other strategies might be a more useful focus of preventive energy).

Summary box: the case for nicotine patches

Setting: How motivated were the patient population of this practice? If they were highly motivated, this might restrict the generalizability of these results.

Subjects: It is important to know how they were selected and what proportion of smokers they represent.

Intervention: The enthusiasm of the nurse might have influenced the result. Is the whole package replicable in settings other than this study?

End-points: The 3-month data were more promising than the 12-month outcome; this is a concern since long-term abstinence is the goal.

Result: The difference between the study groups was statistically significant but the active patch only gave a small absolute additional benefit over placebo. However, that benefit may well be worth having.

Costs: The patches as well as staff time in the short term, which have to be weighed against potential lower rates of smoking-related illness in the future.

Training of staff in health promotion may be needed.

Reflection stop

Try now to reassess this result from the point of view of your own practice – would it be worthwhile systematically prescribing nicotine patches to as many heavy smokers as you could?

SINUS X-RAYS IN GENERAL PRACTICE

Question

What are the implications of the study findings in the light of the College's recommendations? Try answering the question before you read the box and text below. Give yourself 15 minutes to answer the question.

The Royal College of Radiologists have suggested that plain sinus radiography should not be available for GPs and should be requested only by specialists. A paper by Houghton *et al.* (1994) addressed this in a primary care study. All 694 general practitioners in Greater Glasgow were sent a postal questionnaire about their use of sinus X-ray films. 582 doctors replied (84% response) and 448 of these (77%) stated that they requested such films when indicated. The most common reasons cited for these requests were persistent facial pain, frequent attacks of acute sinusitis and responding to patient requests.

Generalization

Setting and subjects

The setting was general practice in one large area, and information was obtained from most of the general practices targeted. There are two points which could be made.

First, such a sample is likely to represent a broad range of individual GP attitudes and practice. In this sense the answers from such a survey are potentially representative of many GPs and can be extrapolated beyond the confines of this particular study.

Second, and in contrast, is the fact that this was done in one geographic area where the local access to sinus radiology, and the quality of the service, might have a profound influence on GP attitudes and their use of the service. It is possible that in other areas with different access to sinus radiology, GPs might have a more restrictive policy with respect to requests anyway. The implications for any particular practice will also depend on their own current practice policy with respect to sinus X-rays.

However, it is likely that the range of reasons for requests will be similar to elsewhere and that the major source of variation will be between individual practitioners regardless of their geographical location.

The intervention

The potential intervention which is being studied is the removal of a resource for general practitioners, namely the opportunity to order a sinus X-ray directly. Since most responders in this survey reported that they would order such films, this is clearly a relevant issue for many general practitioners.

However, the extent to which the results can be extrapolated will need some further information. In particular, the frequency of requests by different practitioners would be crucial. Although most doctors in the sample might order a film at some time, the frequency with which they do it might vary widely. If a few doctors were ordering most of the films, this would have different implications compared with a situation of regular requests from the majority of doctors in the sample.

End-points

If the reasons given for the requests by the GP responders in this study can be generalized as representing GPs' views in general, it is less clear that these reasons are the most important outcomes to consider in drawing out the implications. We would need to be given information about the costs and benefits of performing X-rays for these reasons, for example, the frequency with which important pathologies are identified, how often the X-rays affect management, and whether there are overall benefits for the patients who are X-rayed (including the positive effects of reassurance).

Consequences of introducing the guidelines

For doctors

Since most GPs ordered a sinus X-ray at some time, the first consequence would be that most practices would be affected by such a withdrawal of services.

For patients

These would depend on the further information outlined in End-points above. Specifically:

(a) Would important diagnoses be delayed if persistent facial pain could not be investigated? Would this matter, i.e. would the clinical course of the disease be affected by the delay?
(b) Would the quality of management of recurrent sinusitis in practice be affected if X-rays were not available?

If the answers to these are 'no', then the consequence might be that patients' sinus problems would receive the same quality of care, but without exposure to unnecessary X-rays (which equals radiation, money and time). Alternatively the patients might prove more difficult to manage because of diagnostic uncertainty and their demand for X-rays.

For resources

One consequence of saying only specialists can order X-rays is that all patients who would be referred for an X-ray at present would instead be referred to a specialist (which might mean increased time, cost, and waiting times). If specialists always order an X-ray, then nothing would be gained, and possibly much would be lost.

More information would help to judge this consequence. What proportion of patients referred for X-ray were subsequently sent for specialist opinion? Do those GPs who never ordered sinus X-rays refer more patients to specialists, i.e. in general, is open access sinus radiology saving on specialist referral?

For workload

This might increase if patients need more counselling and information about the costs and benefits of doing X-rays, or if they consult more frequently in the absence of the reassurance of a normal X-ray.

For audit

Audit by individual GPs of their X-ray referrals might help to improve the cost-effectiveness of this type of investigation. It might also soften the impact of any edict to reduce referrals.

For training

Another consequence might be that GPs need to be more skilled in the clinical assessment of sinus symptoms, so that patients would only be referred if they had a high likelihood that specialist investigation and management would actually contribute. An implication of withdrawing radiology might be that GPs, radiologists and clinical consultants would need to draw up agreed guidelines for appropriate hospital referral.

Social and general implications

There might need to be a general shift in the 'X-ray' culture to reduce the element of patient demand for such a service. Consultants need to be involved in this, for whilst they may withdraw a GP service because of its expense, they may use it themselves in an equally irrational manner (e.g. X-ray all referrals), which is only less expensive because the GPs are forced to do further selection in terms of whom they send to hospital.

More research into the natural history of persistent facial pain and recurrent sinusitis would help rational decision-making in general practice.

Summary box: sinus X-rays

Setting: One specific geographical area. Access to and the quality of the X-ray service are likely to influence result.

Subjects: It is likely that a broad range of GP opinion was included.

Intervention: The effect of removing direct access would depend on the frequency of requests by different GPs.

End-points: Reassurance of patients is a valid end-point. How often do X-ray results influence management?

Consequences: Restriction of GPs freedom, possibility of delay in diagnosis or increase in referrals. Education and guidelines about the assessment of facial pain may be needed. It may be hard to alter patients' health beliefs about the importance of X-rays.

Reflection stop

X-rays in practice

- Consider the implications of this study for your own practice.
- What would you rather have: open access radiology, fast-track referral to the specialist, better clinical knowledge about sinusitis?
- Consider other situations where there are the same dilemmas, such as X-rays for low back pain, Doppler imaging of carotid arteries.
- List the arguments for and against your preferred service.

PNEUMATIC OTOSCOPY IN GENERAL PRACTICE

Question

Read the study title and summary below, adapted from de Melker (1993). Consider the implications for general practice. What additional information would you find helpful before introducing pneumatic otoscopy into your practice?

Title: Evaluation of the diagnostic value of pneumatic otoscopy in primary care using the results of tympanometry as a reference standard.

Summary: The aim of this study was to determine the value of pneumatic otoscopy in diagnosing otitis media with effusion in primary care. Pneumatic otoscopy was carried out for 111 children aged one to 16 years and the results obtained compared with those obtained from tympanometry. The children were those who attended for a regular ear nose and throat check up in the health centre of a school for the deaf during the period November 1989 to January 1990. Pneumatic otoscopy and tympanometry were carried out by a trained ear, nose and throat nurse. The results of tympanometry were evaluated independently of the otoscopic findings. In the population examined the predictive values of positive and negative results of pneumatic otoscopy for diagnosing effusion were high; the sensitivity was low.

It was concluded that pneumatic otoscopy carried out by an experienced health care worker is of high diagnostic value when compared with the results of tympanometry. Pneumatic otoscopy can improve the diagnostic capabilities of general practitioners and other primary care workers with regard to otitis media with effusion.

Generalization

Aims, setting and subjects

The title makes clear that the diagnostic value of pneumatic otoscopy in primary care is to be evaluated. It is unclear from the abstract whether the setting and the subjects were typical of those children in primary care who would be candidates for a diagnosis of otitis media with effusion. There are a number of reasons for supposing that they were not typical: they were attending for a regular ENT check-up, they were attending the health centre of a school for the deaf (although it is not stated whether they themselves were pupils of the school), the age range was unusually broad compared with the important ages for this problem in primary care.

So there is a question as to whether the subjects and the setting can be generalized to primary care patients needing a diagnosis of otitis media.

Having made that general point, you should then go on to ask 'Does it matter?'. As we said earlier in the chapter, beware of rejecting a study because it was not done on a typical set of primary care patients. You must look at the purpose of the study. It was to establish the value of pneumatic otoscopy in diagnosing effusion in primary care. There are two important points:

1 Given that aim, some concern remains. The 'value' of pneumatic otoscopy will include lots of aspects, such as the practicality of doing the examination in a primary care setting, which this study might not be able to answer if the setting and subjects were not typical of those seen in primary care.
2 The main comparison of the study however (how does otoscopy perform against tympanometry as a gold standard?) does not

necessarily need to be performed in primary care to be relevant to primary care. In later chapters we will consider sensitivity and specificity in detail. For the moment, note that evaluating whether a test can identify a high proportion of those who have the disease (sensitivity) and rule out a high proportion of those without the disease (specificity) does not depend very strongly on what group of patients you choose to study.

However, a much more important measure of the performance of a diagnostic test in primary care settings is its positive predictive value – if I test positive, how likely am I to have the disease? A general rule that is useful to remember is that predictive value is much higher when estimated in groups of patients where the disease is common. So if this group had a high prevalence of effusion on tympanometry because they were a group of children with chronic hearing problems, then the predictive value of otoscopy will be higher than if it were estimated in a group of children in primary care who had a lower prevalence of effusion than the group studied here.

From the abstract we can make no judgement on whether the predictive value can be generalized to the primary care setting or to the population in primary care who might be referred for otoscopy.

The intervention

This is pneumatic otoscopy, with a gold standard intervention of tympanometry. Even if you know nothing about either of these tests, you can ask some questions about their relevance to primary care:

- How practical is otoscopy?
- Does it need a specialist nurse?
- How long does it take?
- How expensive is the equipment?
- Could it be performed in the average general practice?

And why is it being tested for its utility in primary care – is it more relevant to that setting than tympanometry, i.e. more practical, quicker, cheaper, needing less specialized training? (If the answers to these questions are 'no', then why not assess the value of tympanometry itself for its applicability in primary care?)

Finally, why pneumatic otoscopy rather than ordinary otoscopy or a whisper test? We need further information on whether this proposed test had a better predictive value than simpler procedures when they were tested against tympanometry.

The outcomes

The title makes the point of the study very clear – to judge how well otoscopy performs against tympanometry. However, in considering the wider implications of a study, it is entirely reasonable to get beyond the immediate purpose of the investigation, and consider the general relevance of these tests for primary care. We need more information on the value of tympanometric diagnosis of effusion to judge this – does it alter practice? Would it affect referral rates and improve the management of children we suspect of having effusion? or would we wish to get a specialist opinion on children whom we or the parents suspect of having troublesome deafness? The relevance of the otoscopic test to primary care is dependent on knowing the exact value and place in primary care of the gold standard (tympanometry) chosen for the study.

The result

The extent to which the high predictive value can be generalized is partly dependent on the points raised in the section on intervention above. However, it is also dependent on seeing the actual figures – we need more details than are provided in the abstract. In brief, we want to know how many in the study population had effusions according to the gold standard, what proportion of these were picked up by otoscopy, and what proportion were missed by otoscopy. The importance of the actual results can then be judged.

Consequences

Costs

What are the costs of equipment, maintenance, and personnel, and who would bear them? In particular the critical question is whether a dedicated trained nurse would be needed or could members of the practice team perform the test? If the former, what are the costs and the workload? If the latter, there may be a need to educate the doctors or practice nurses or health visitors, and to monitor their performance.

Referrals

If the test was used when effusion was suspected, one consequence might be that the number of confident diagnoses of effusion would increase and there might be more referrals to specialists.

Screening or diagnostic test?

General practitioners might feel more and more inclined to use the test as a screening instrument rather than as a diagnostic tool for individuals in whom there is a high suspicion that an effusion is present. So, for example, all children who present with acute otitis media might be asked to return a month later for the test. Such strategies can often develop in the context of primary care (think of blood pressure measurement, peak flow measurement, urinalysis) and they may be very reasonable, but the consequences of using such a test as a screening tool need to be thought through. Consider workload again as well as the numbers who might be diagnosed as having some abnormality – how should they be managed and has the practice got the resources to cope? Are abnormalities clear-cut or are there lots of borderlines? (Think of the problems that borderline hypertension can cause in terms of decisions to treat.)

Potential for organized primary care follow-up

A positive consequence might be that the management of suspected deafness and the follow-up of acute otitis media could be organized in a formal fashion with the trained nurse responsible for it, rather than relying on haphazard and variable follow-up times or referrals. Management of these problems could become a primary care team issue, focused on an otoscopy clinic.

Summary box: pneumatic otoscopy in general practice

Aim: Clearly stated in title.

Subjects: It is unclear whether they have chronic hearing problems; if so, the predictive value of the screening test is unlikely to be generalizable to a primary care population.

> **Intervention**: How much training is needed and how practical is it really? Why not use tympanometry itself?
>
> **End-points**: Does diagnosis of effusion alter management?
>
> **Result**: How many children had effusions and what proportion were picked up by pneumatic otoscopy?
>
> **Costs**: Staff time and training plus equipment.
>
> **Referrals**: It is unclear whether this should be a screening test for all children presenting in primary care with suspected serous otitis media; if so the referral rate to secondary care is likely to go up.
>
> **Follow-up** of acute otitis media might be more systematic if this facility were available: i.e. it might be applied to a selected group.

PREVENTING DIABETIC COMPLICATIONS

Question

Read the summary below, and then write short notes on the implications for diabetes care in British general practice. Taken from the Diabetes Control and Complications Trial Research Group (1993).

> **Title**: The effect of intensive treatment of diabetes on the development and progression of long-term complications in insulin-dependent diabetes mellitus.
>
> **Abstract**
>
> *Background*: Long-term microvascular and neurologic complications cause major morbidity and mortality in patients with insulin-dependent diabetes mellitus (IDDM). We examined whether intensive treatment with the goal of maintaining blood glucose concentrations close to the normal range could decrease the frequency and severity of these complications.

Methods: A total of 1441 patients with IDDM – 726 with no retinopathy at baseline (the primary prevention cohort) and 715 with mild retinopathy (the secondary intervention cohort) – were randomly assigned to intensive therapy administered either with an external insulin pump or by three or more daily insulin injections and guided by frequent blood glucose monitoring or to conventional therapy with one or two daily insulin injections. The patients were followed for a mean of 6.5 years, and the appearance and progression of retinopathy and other complications were assessed regularly.

Results: In the primary prevention cohort, intensive therapy reduced the adjusted mean risk for the development of retinopathy by 76% (95% confidence interval, 62 to 85%), as compared with conventional therapy. In the secondary intervention cohort, intensive therapy slowed the progression of retinopathy by 54% (95% confidence interval, 39 to 66%) and reduced the development of proliferative or severe non-proliferative retinopathy by 47% (95% confidence interval, 14 to 67%). In the two cohorts combined, intensive therapy reduced the occurrence of microalbuminuria (urinary albumin excretion of >40 mg per 24 hours) by 39% (95% confidence interval, 21 to 52%), that of albuminuria (urinary albumin excretion of >300 mg per 24 hours) by 54% (95% confidence interval, 19 to 74%), and that of clinical neuropathy by 60% (95% confidence interval, 38 to 74%). The chief adverse event associated with intensive therapy was a two-to-threefold increase in severe hypoglycaemia.

Conclusions: Intensive therapy effectively delays the onset and slows the progression of diabetic retinopathy, nephropathy, and neuropathy in patients with IDDM.

Suggested answer

Design

This was a randomized controlled trial in insulin-dependent diabetics involving clearly defined patient groups. The results are thus potentially generalizable to diabetics in the UK.

Intensity of care and reduction of complications

It is likely that only a very small minority of patients in the UK are receiving the intensity of care described for the active intervention group. If the results are reliable, the first implication is that changes in diabetic care could prevent and slow down the current level of complications in insulin-dependent diabetics. The potential for improvement in the incidence of retinopathy, nephropathy and neuropathy looks to be considerable.

Process of care: cost, workload, acceptability

The implications must take account of the processes involved in achieving the reductions seen in this trial. The provision of a pump, or an increased regularity of insulin injections, together with the need for frequent blood glucose monitoring, have many potential implications for practice in the UK: additional costs, additional workload for health care professionals in training and supervising, patient acceptability, patient compliance. To the extent that any of these would have a significant effect in reducing the uptake or delivery of intensive therapy, then the overall effect of the intervention would be less than that seen in the trial. Being in a trial is a highly motivating process and this may influence the result. Such an effect is sometimes referred to as the 'Hawthorne effect'.

Large size of intervention

Against this must be weighed the fact that the changes in relative terms were quite large, so that even if a less efficient regime was introduced or even if there were a considerable number of patients who refused or did not wish to adhere to the regime, it still might have an impact on the occurrence of diabetic complications. One implication might be that more modest but useful benefits might emerge even if the trial protocol could not be put into practice universally in the UK.

Side effects of treatment

Of more concern is the increase in severe hypoglycaemia. Under the highly controlled conditions which a trial demands, the published incidence of hypoglycaemic events is likely to represent the most optimistic situation. Putting the regime into practice in the real world is likely to mean many more such events, and probably more serious outcomes. Since hypoglycaemia kills, the universal adoption of this approach might result in unacceptable mortality rates – more costs than benefits, in fact.

Patient autonomy

The need for careful and highly controlled intervention also goes against the general approach to diabetics which encourages their independence and self-monitoring. Any attempt to introduce this regime in the UK would need to be slow, in chosen patient groups, and with careful monitoring of effects.

Reflection stop

Consider the regime described in this study in relation to the diabetic patients for whom you care.

- What proportion might be eligible for such a regime?
- How many might wish to try it?
- Have you concerns about introducing it even for the minority of diabetics who would like to try it?
- Does it fit with your general ideas about diabetic control, and the risks and benefits of such intensive regimes?
- What changes and resources might be demanded of your own practice to institute such a regime?

REFERENCES

Colledge, N.R., Barr-Hamilton, R.M., Lewis, S.J., Sellar, R.J., and Wilson, J.A. (1996) Evaluation of investigations to diagnose the cause of dizziness in elderly people: a community based controlled study. *British Medical Journal*, **313**, 788–92.

de Melker, R.A. (1993) Evaluation of the diagnostic value of pneumatic otoscopy in primary care using the results of typanometry as a reference standard. *British Journal of General Practice*, **43**, 22–4.

Diabetes Control and Complications Trial Research Group, (1993) The effect of intensive treatment of diabetes on the development and progession of long-term complications in insulin-dependent diabetes mellitus. *New England Journal of Medicine*, **329**, 977–86.

Houghton, D.J., Aitchison, F.A., Wilkinson, L., and Wilson, J.A. (1994) Use of sinus Xray films by general practitioners, *British Medical Journal*, **308**, 1608–9.

ICRF General Practice Research Group. (1994) Randomised trial of nicotine patches in general practice: results at one year. *British Medical Journal*, **308**, 1476–7.

Little, P., Williamson, I., Warner, G., Gould, C., Gantley, M., and Kinmonth, A.L. (1997) Open randomised trial of prescribing strategies in managing sore throat. *British Medical Journal*, **314**, 722–7.

MacGregor, G.A., Markandu, N.D., Sagnella, G.A., Singer, D.R.J., and Cappuccio, F.P. (1989) Double-blind study of three sodium intakes and long-term effects of sodium restriction in essential hypertension. *Lancet*, **(ii)**, 1244–7.

Shvartzman, P., Tabenkin, H., Rosentzwalg, A., and Dolginov, F. (1993) Treatment of streptococcal pharyngitis with amoxycillin once a day. *British Medical Journal*, **306**, 1170–2.

7

Making sense of screening

A patient presents with low back pain. You embark on a brief series of questions. When did it start? What appeared to bring it on? Any problems in the legs? Feel quite well otherwise?

Your view of the low back pain of

> a 25-year-old man, perfectly fit, whose symptom started after an unusually long car journey 5 days ago, and who has no radiating symptoms in his legs,

will be different to your view of the low back pain in

> a 75-year-old lady, who has been losing weight and feeling generally unwell for 3 months and whose problem came on gradually during that time and is now nagging and persistent throughout the day.

The history-taking has pushed these two patients into two different categories of diagnostic 'probability'. The probability of any new episode of low back pain being relatively benign and likely to settle is high anyway. In the man's case, his age and his history makes this conclusion even more likely. In the woman's case, however, her age and her history raises the probability of a serious problem (tumour, infection, osteoporotic fracture) high enough to justify further action.

The remit of primary care includes much more than such 'presenting symptom medicine'. For example, the fact that most people with hypertension do not have symptoms provides a reason to check blood pressures routinely. Every time a practice nurse checks a blood pressure in a fit person for the first time, he or she is conducting a **screening test**: looking for evidence of disease in a person with no symptoms.

In some ways screening may seem to be fundamentally different from diagnosis because disease is looked for in individuals who do not have symptoms. But the process is similar: asking questions, using physical examinations or applying a test. The key difference is that when used for screening, these approaches are being used in a group of patients who are less likely to have the condition than a group with characteristic symptoms. This is important when symptoms are a poor guide to diagnosis or represent too late a manifestation of the problem for remedial or therapeutic action.

> Some individuals have a higher probability of developing or having colon cancer than the general population. Screening (whether on the basis of genes, lifestyle or testing for pathology before symptoms start) is a matter of moving the start of the diagnostic process back to a point earlier than the usual 'visit the doctor with a symptom'.

Whether or not this is worthwhile will depend on many things, but the outcome for the patient needs to be better than waiting for symptoms to present. (Outcome includes quality of life as well as delayed death.)

The 'classical' screening test for a disease involves a simple manoeuvre that can be applied to a group of subjects in order to identify those individuals who are more likely than the rest to have the disease. The true diagnosis is established by a 'gold standard'.

> Screening for breast cancer is by mammography. Women who have a positive mammogram have a needle biopsy to establish the 'true' diagnosis.

It would be impractical, expensive and unacceptable to use needle biopsy to screen large numbers of women for breast cancer. Once mammography has narrowed the field down to a small number of women, it becomes acceptable and affordable to use needle biopsy.

A gold standard might still be impractical to use in a group which has been screened.

> Screening children for serous otitis media using a 'whisper' test in primary care does not narrow down the field of likely candidates with sufficient certainty to be followed by aspiration of the middle ear. Instead an intermediate 'reference' standard is used, such as tympanometry.

In this chapter we will use the term 'gold standard' to mean any chosen indicator of the 'true' diagnosis, however arbitrary it may be.

Summary box: useful things to know about screening

1 The different strategies of preventive health.
2 The established criteria for an effective screening test.
3 The meaning of terms used to evaluate the screening procedure itself: sensitivity, specificity, predictive value.
4 That diagnosis and screening are not separate categories but on a continuum related to how frequently a disease occurs in the population.
5 That screening jargon applies equally well to diagnostic testing.

TEST YOURSELF: PREVENTION

Question

Before reading further, write a short summary of what you understand by the terms primary, secondary and tertiary prevention. Then continue.

THREE STRATEGIES FOR PREVENTION

There are three main strategies for preventing disease or the consequences of disease. (Not everyone uses the same terminology here: if your definitions are very different, see the note below.)

Primary prevention

This is the broad sweep approach. It targets society as a whole. Examples include vaccination and legislation to enforce behavioural change such as the wearing of seat belts or raising the taxes on cigarettes. This is the traditional public health approach and does not involve the targeting of individuals.

Secondary prevention

By contrast secondary prevention does identify individuals, either people who are at increased risk of developing disease or people who have an early stage of a disease which can be treated effectively. The latter is 'classical screening', as typified by the breast cancer screening programme. The former is what often happens in primary care – identifying those who smoke, are overweight, or have raised blood pressure, or older people who are at risk of falling or children who are at risk of abuse.

Secondary prevention can target large groups at specific times (breast or cervical cancer screening, invitations to attend the surgery for a check of blood pressure) or take place opportunistically when the patient is attending for another reason (registration medicals, blood pressure checks in routine surgeries).

Tertiary prevention

This is not about preventing the onset of disease, but about reducing the burden, consequences or recurrence of disease. For example, low back pain is a common problem, but most disability occurs in the chronic cases. Effective treatment of acute cases may reduce the incidence of chronicity. This is tertiary prevention. Another target for such prevention would be effective management of chronic low back pain to reduce disability and handicap.

Note: Some clinicians (and publications such as the British National Formulary) largely ignore the public health approach and refer to primary prevention as the targeting of high-risk individuals before they develop a disease and secondary prevention as the prevention of further disease in someone who already has the condition. So primary prevention of coronary heart disease might mean identifying and treating individuals with familial hyperlipidaemia. Secondary prevention of myocardial infarction would include treatment with aspirin for those with angina or a previous myocardial infarct. So if you use these terms, make it clear exactly what you mean.

TEST YOURSELF: SCREENING PRINCIPLES

CRITERIA FOR AN EFFECTIVE SCREENING PROGRAMME

Question

Before you say, 'Oh no, not Wilson's criteria again . . .', write a list of as many of Wilson's criteria as you can remember (Wilson, 1976). Then read our mnemonic (which summarizes the main criteria) in the Box 7.1.

Box 7.1 Wilson's criteria: TRAP WILSON

Four main points

T   Treatable condition
R   Resources for screening and treatment
A   Activity should be continuous process
    Audit cycle must be continued
P   Protocols needed: clear policy of when to treat

Plus six other criteria

W   Worthwhile (cost vs benefit)
I   Important to individual and community
L   Latent phase exists
S   Suitable and acceptable test
O   Outcome improved by early detection
N   Natural history well understood

Mant and Fowler

If you find Wilson's criteria rather cumbersome or difficult to remember, there is a paper which summarizes screening from the primary care perspective (Mant and Fowler, 1990). The authors propose a list of criteria which emphasize two factors of crucial importance to GPs: firstly, the implications of false alarms and secondly, ways to minimize anxiety and distress.

There is an explicit ethical responsibility to each individual being screened to ensure that the process of screening is more likely to benefit than harm. The Box 7.2 summarizes the Mant and Fowler criteria.

Box 7.2 Mant and Fowler: criteria for screening.

Mass screening in general practice

'Enthusiasm to do good is simply not enough.' Minimum criteria include:

1 Carefully defined protocols
2 Availability of effective treatment
3 Implications of false alarms
4 Workload implications manageable
5 Audit methods planned
6 Ethical implications considered

Ethical issues

● Aim for more benefit than harm for each patient
● Inform patients of balance of risk and benefit
● Minimize false reassurance and false alarms
● Ensure effective intervention
● Audit follow-up

DIAGNOSIS OR SCREENING?

Many research-based articles attempt to provide evidence that one route to diagnosis is better than another. The focus of such articles might be an item of clinical history or examination or it might be a new piece of technology to be introduced into practice. Is it to be used for screening or diagnosis?

For this section, we are going to use the example from the previous chapter on the possibility of introducing a new test for glue ear into primary care (pneumatic otoscopy). The abstract described a comparison of this test, applied by a trained nurse, with results obtained from typanometry (de Melker, 1993).

> Assume, for example, that there was no controversy over the management of established glue ear and that there was good evidence that treatment is effective in preventing continuing deafness, associated behavioural difficulties and later problems of learning and communication.
>
> These are some of the possibilities for the new test:
>
> 1 Screen all children up to 7 years old, for example, whether they have symptoms or not.
> 2 Screen all children presenting with an upper respiratory infection.
> 3 Screen all children with acute otitis media 6 weeks after the acute event.
> 4 Screen only those in whom parents or teachers report deafness or behaviour problems.
> 5 Screen only those with deafness and an abnormal tympanic membrane on otoscopy.

The distinction between diagnosis and screening is disappearing as we consider these possibilities. The first option might be regarded as classic screening and the last option as a diagnostic test, but what about the examples in between? What is happening?

The important point is the population you start with. If you choose option (1) and screen all children, then there is a relatively low probability of finding it, because there will be lots of children who do not have it. The advantage might be in identifying children with glue ear who have not presented with obvious symptoms. This is 'classical screening'. It might be justified if there was evidence of advantage in identifying and treating such apparently asymptomatic children.

In practice a more selective application of the new test is likely. This means identifying children with a higher probability of having glue ear compared to others in a given age range. Children attending with repeated upper respiratory infections might be such a group. Testing children after acute otitis media might narrow things further or we could confine our attention to children in whom glue ear was suspected on the basis of a combination of symptoms and otoscopic findings. Each group is progressively more select with a correspondingly higher probability of glue ear.

At each step along this pathway of increasing selectivity, some children with glue ear will be excluded from the new test (those without symptoms, for example, when choosing option (2) instead of option (1) or those without otoscopic abnormalities when choosing (5) instead of (4)). The advantage is that fewer children are tested who do not have the disease.

There are a number of issues specific to whole population screening, but one of them is practical. How many children could we test with available time, money and resources? Any decision about how to use the new test will need to balance these costs and benefits.

The general point is that any 'test' which aims to bring us nearer to a diagnosis – be it a simple question to the patient or the latest sophisticated imaging test – does not take place in a vacuum. How well a test performs depends on the population to which it is applied.

Jargon corner

Diagnosis or screening?

This is an artificial distinction.

Faced with a paper about a new test – whether it is a clinical sign or an imaging machine – ask:

● In what population has it been studied?
● To what population is it to be applied?

DESCRIBING THE PERFORMANCE OF A TEST

There are certain formal ways to describe and quantify diagnostic procedures, and it is useful to know these.

Sensitivity

Regardless of the population group studied, we will assume that there are a certain number of people who truly have the condition being studied. The sensitivity of a test indicates the proportion or percentage of these 'true' cases which the test will correctly identify. In the example quoted above, the test under scrutiny is pneumatic otoscopy. The gold standard which establishes the 'true' diagnosis of glue ear is tympanometry.

> The sensitivity of the test = the proportion of cases of glue ear defined by tympanometry which will be identified correctly by pneumatic otoscopy.

Note two things about this:

a The sensitivity is not altered by changing the population studied, as long as the same disease is being considered.

> Glue ear, defined by tympanometry, will be more common in a group of 5 year olds presenting to the GP with deafness and earache than in a random sample of all 5 year olds in the same practice. The *proportion* of cases which pneumatic otoscopy would identify correctly (the sensitivity) will be similar in these two situations.

b The sensitivity of a test is not an absolute figure – it is entirely dependent on the 'gold standard' chosen. In this example tympanometry was stated explicitly to be the standard against which pneumatic otoscopy was to be judged, and that is fine and clear. However, 'glue ear established by tympanometry' is a different entity to 'glue ear diagnosed by the surgical drainage of infected or inflamed fluid from the middle ear'. The choice of gold standard is influenced by 'current state of knowledge' and the question being addressed by the study.

In this case a practice-based diagnosis is being investigated as a practical alternative to referral for tympanometry, so using the latter as the gold standard by which to judge the new test's performance is reasonable. Some writers would use the term 'reference standard' for a test like tympanometry when there is a defining 'gold standard' like surgical detection of middle ear fluid.

Specificity

Since the gold standard identifies a group of people who 'truly' have the condition, it also must define those who do *not* have it. The specificity of the test is the proportion correctly identified as free of the disease out of all those who are 'truly' free of it.

Once again, this proportion is unaffected by the population in whom the study is being carried out or to whom it is intended to apply. Although the prevalence of normal middle ears in a random sample of 5 year olds is higher than in children with earache and deafness, the *proportion* of 'true' normals correctly identified by the new test is going to be the same in both situations.

Jargon corner

Sensitivity tells us what proportion of gold standard positives our test correctly identifies, and **specificity** tells us what proportion of gold standard negatives it correctly labels. Both are:

- **Dependent** on the choice of gold standard, but usually
- **Independent** of the prevalence of the condition.

Predictive value

So why all this fuss about being clear in what population the study has been done, if sensitivity and specificity do not depend on how rare or common the disease is?

The reason can be illustrated by considering once again the example of glue ear (de Melker, 1993).

Let us suppose that 5% of children screened at random aged 5 years have tympanometry diagnosed glue ear, but that 20% of children presenting with earache and deafness have it. In each situation let us suppose that the sensitivity of pneumatic otoscopy in identifying these cases was 75%, and that specificity was 90%.

If 1000 symptomatic children were studied, the number with 'true' disease would be 200 (i.e. 20% of the total); 150 (75%) of these would be correctly identified by pneumatic otoscopy and 50 would be missed (false negatives).

Table 7.1 Symptomatic children

	Tympanometry positive	Tympanometry negative	Total
Pneumatic positive	150	80	230
Pneumatic negative	50	720	770
Total	200	800	1000

The number who 'truly' do not have the disease would be 800 (80% of the total); 720 (90%) of these would be correctly identified by the new test as having no glue ear which means that 80 would be incorrectly labelled as positives (false positives). Table 7.1 summarizes these figures.

So a total of 230 children (150 plus 80) would test positive, of whom 150 'truly' have the condition as judged by tympanometry.

In this table the sensitivity (150/200) = 75%, the specificity (720/800) = 90%, the positive predictive value (150/230) = 65%.

If 1000 randomly sampled children were studied, the number with 'true' disease would be 50 (5% of the total); 38 (75%) of these would be correctly identified by pneumatic otoscopy (12 would be missed: false negatives). The number who 'truly' do not have the disease would be 950 (95% of the total); 855 (90%) of these would be correctly identified by the new test as having no glue ear which means that 95 would be incorrectly labelled as positives. So in total 133 (38 plus 95) children would test positive, of whom only 38

Table 7.2 Random sample of asymptomatic children

	Tympanometry positive	Tympanometry negative	Total
Pneumatic positive	38	95	133
Pneumatic negative	12	855	867
Total	50	950	1000

'truly' have the condition as judged by tympanometry. This situation is summarized in Table 7.2.

This time the sensitivity (38/50) = 75%, specificity (855/950) = 90%, and positive predictive value (38/133) = 29%.

Jargon corner

People who test positive and do have 'gold standard' disease are called **true positives**; those who test negative and this is confirmed by the 'gold standard' are termed **true negatives**. Those whom the test incorrectly labels as diseased or not diseased are false positives and negatives respectively.

Changing the prevalence of 'true' disease, as in the examples above, by changing the population in which the prevalence is measured, has altered the **predictive value** of the test.

The **positive predictive value** of a test is the proportion of all those who test positive who truly have the disease (i.e. gold standard positives).

The **negative predictive value** of a test is the proportion of all those who test negative who are true negatives.

Although sensitivity and specificity are constant in the two situations considered above, the proportion of true positives and true negatives among all those whom the test is identifying has altered. In other words predictive values alter according to the prevalence of gold standard disease in the population under review.

Jargon corner

Positive predictive value is the proportion of all those testing positive who have the 'gold standard' disease or condition being screened for. It varies with the true prevalence of disease in the population being screened.

In the examples above, the positive predictive value in the symptomatic population is 65% (150/230), compared with 29% (38/133) in the randomly sampled group. What has happened is that the number of false positives has swamped the number of true positives in the randomly sampled group, an important issue when considering the pros and cons of screening in the general population. The lower prevalence means that the effects of a less than 100% specificity get magnified, because a much larger proportion of the population do not in reality have disease.

So the positive predictive value gives a guide to the balance between true positives and false positives. False positives can create unjustified anxiety for patients as well as enormous workload implications for both primary and secondary care. This balance between true and false positives is dependent on the prevalence of the disease being sought and is a very important measure of the usefulness of a screening test. The take home message is that the positive predictive value must be calculated for the situation in which the test is to be used.

The negative predictive value in the symptomatic children is 94% (720 true negatives out of a total of 770 who tested negative), compared with 99% (855 true negatives out of a total of 867 testing negative) in the randomly sampled group. The corollary of the low prevalence is that the number of false negatives is small compared with all those who test negative.

This explains why context is crucial when judging the performance of any test. What is an efficient and useful test in a hospital clinic can be a monster when applied to the population attending primary care or to the community at large. The number of false labels can soon outflank the number of correct labels. Rather than viewing it as a simple dichotomy between diagnosis in a high prevalence setting versus screening in a low prevalence setting, we should regard it as a continuum.

So let us return to our example: how should we identify glue ear? Imagine the process of identification broken down into stages:

a Firstly we could identify all children aged 0–7 years in the practice.
b Next we could wait for them to present with symptoms. Those with acute otitis media will be followed up. (FIRST stage of testing: select a simple method of identifying an at-risk group –

those who present with symptoms. PROBLEM: you miss the asymptomatic or unpresented glue ears.)

c Leave them for 4 weeks. (SECOND stage of testing: select a simple method of excluding those who get better anyway and would not require further treatment. PROBLEM: as for stage one above.)

d Test them with a whisper test and routine visualization of the drum. (THIRD stage of testing: define the group to have special investigation by means of simple clinical procedures. PROBLEM: how good are these simple procedures at identifying likely glue ear? If they have little additional value over the second stage, then this stage will either be of no benefit or actually be harmful – because it will have spuriously excluded those at risk – and a better option might be to investigate all children who present with acute otitis media regardless of the subsequent clinical findings. In other words, the predictive values need to be known for each step in the process.)

e Carry out pneumatic otoscopy. (FOURTH stage, the new test. PROBLEM: even if it performs well compared with the gold standard, at this stage you might ask why not go straight for the gold standard? Here come in questions of cost and practicality, and whether you will actually reduce the number of referrals for tympanometry or not.)

f Do tympanometry. (FIFTH stage, definitive diagnosis. PROBLEM: Is there any point in doing it, if the previous stage has defined a group sufficiently narrowly that surgical treatment is likely to help any way?)

g Treatment. (Evidence for efficacy?)

The final stage of thinking through this is to arrive at the idea of likelihoods. Each stage of the process should increase the likelihood of reaching a diagnosis. So the utility or usefulness of applying a diagnostic test at any particular stage should be assessed relative to the prior likelihood of the group having the disease in question, and to the change in that likelihood that you achieve by doing the test. This can be summarized by a statistic called the **likelihood ratio**, which you can find described in textbooks of clinical epidemiology, such as Sackett *et al.* (1997). If the test makes little difference, then that step in the diagnostic process is of questionable value.

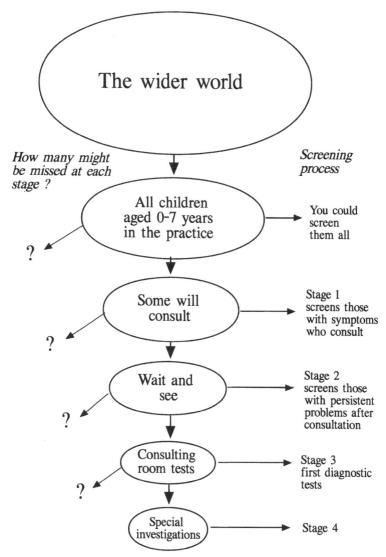

Figure 7.1 Potential stages for screening or diagnosing glue ear.

This whole process has also to take into account the practicality, the cost and the ability to provide the next step and an effective treatment at the end of the process.

This pathway and the choices it involves is summarized in Figure 7.1.

A QUICK APPROACH TO SCREENING TEST STATISTICS

Screening tests range from the classical type of diagnostic test (e.g. urine strips for glucose as a test for diabetes) to the use of an item of history or examination as a 'screen' for disease (e.g. asking parents about their child's hearing as an initial screen for chronic serous otitis media).

Box 7.3 A 5-step approach to making sense of screening test results.

1 Identify the test and gold standard.
2 Construct a '2×2' table putting gold standard results in the columns and test results in the rows.
3 Note the population being studied and the true disease prevalence.
4 Calculate sensitivity and specificity from the columns of your table.
5 Calculate predictive values from the rows of your table.

We can now apply the 5-step approach to a study of the use of stick tests for nitrites and esterase in urine samples as a method of screening for urinary infection (adapted from Woodward and Griffiths (1993)).

In this paper, the authors introduce the topic as follows:

> Urinary tract infections are common in infancy and childhood and may indicate an underlying urological problem requiring treatment. The standard method for the diagnosis of urinary tract infection remains the microscopic examination and quantitative culture of a clean catch specimen of urine, but recently a dipstick has become available that tests for two markers of infection – leucocyte esterase and nitrites. Leucocyte esterase is an enzyme from neutrophils not normally found in urine and is a marker of pyuria. Almost all urinary pathogens reduce nitrates to nitrites except for certain pseudomonads and group B streptococci.

The dipsticks have been tested extensively in adults but there are few reports of their use in children. Wiggelinkhuizen *et al.* (1988) compared dipstick testing with formal urine analysis of 11 137 children and concluded that the dipsticks were a reliable screening technique. Other groups have also recommended that dipsticks be used instead of urine analysis for rapid screening of children for urinary tract infection since negative results for leucocyte esterase and nitrites indicated the absence of infection. The routine use of dipsticks for screening children's urine is not widespread in the United Kingdom, and so we have retested them to determine whether they should be adopted for primary screening.

The results, summarized and adapted from the paper, were as follows:

Between November 1992 and January 1993 we tested 133 urine samples with the dipsticks (Multistix 10SG, Bayer, Newbury) in our paediatric surgical department. We did not alter our pre-existing criteria for the selection of patients for urine testing: most were children with acute abdominal pain, whose urine was routinely tested. Their mean age was 8.1 years (range 1 month to 15 years), and 71 (53%) were girls. About 86% of the urine samples were taken mid-stream with the rest from a bag or catheter. A positive result was recorded if more than a trace of leucocyte esterase was detected or if any colour change for nitrites occurred.

We detected 12 urinary tract infections based on criteria of >20 white blood cells per microlitre and $>10^5$ organisms per litre of a pure culture. Ten of these were positive for both leucocyte esterase and nitrites and two had tested negative. The other 121 samples were negative on culture and none of these had registered positive for leucocyte esterase or nitrites.

The 5-step approach

(i) **Identify the test and gold standard**
Two screening tests: nitrite test and esterase test.
Gold standard: urine bacteriological culture.

(ii)   **Construct a 2×2 table**
Gold standards in the columns, test results in the rows.

		Gold standard	
		Positive	Negative
Screening test	Positive	A True positive	B False positive
	Negative	C False negative	D True negative

If we now add up the numbers in the boxes, we can insert the marginal values (which are, of course, the values in the margin!).

		Gold standard		
		Positive	Negative	
Screening test	Positive	A True positive	B False positive	A + B
	Negative	C False negative	D True negative	C + D
		A + C	B + D	A + B + C + D

Filling in the values from the urine testing example:

		Microbiology		
		Positive	Negative	
Dipstick	Positive	10	0	10
	Negative	2	121	123
		12	121	133

(iii) **Note the population being studied and the true disease prevalence**

Is the population being studied the same as the population on which you would use the test in your practice? This is a judgement based on the description of the setting and the patients studied. But you can get some help from the bottom row of totals. This tells you the prevalence of true disease (i.e. the proportion of gold standard positives) in this population.

The prevalence of microbiologically cultured positive urines in this study was 12/133 = 9%.

(iv) **Calculate sensitivity and specificity**

Sensitivity and specificity are all about the proportion with and without true disease (proportion of gold standard positives and negatives) detected correctly by the screening test. So for sensitivity and specificity think gold standards and so think columns from your table.

In this example, the sensitivity of the dipstick tests refers to the proportion of all patients diagnosed with a urine infection by microbiological culture who had both markers positive in the dipstick test. This was 10/12 = 83%.

For specificity, read down the column of gold standard negatives. It is the proportion of all urine samples with no culture on microbiology which had been negative to both dipstick tests. This was 121/121 = 100%.

Note that sensitivity and specificity are calculated without crossing the line between columns. These figures remain constant regardless of the prevalence of gold standard positives in the population being studied.

(v) **Calculate predictive values**

For predictive values, think tests and so think rows from your table.

For positive predictive value, look across the first row to calculate the proportion of all positive tests which were subsequently shown to be positive gold standards ('true positives'). The positive predictive value of the dipstick test refers to the proportion of all urines with both markers positive which were subsequently found to have positive bacteriological cultures. This was 10/10 = 100%.

For negative predictive value, look across the second row to calculate the proportion of all negative tests which were subsequently shown to be negative gold standards ('true negatives'). The negative predictive value of the dipstick test refers to the proportion of all urines with both markers negative which were subsequently found to have negative bacteriological cultures. This was 121/123 = 98%.

Note that you have crossed columns in calculating predictive values. The importance of this is that predictive values will change as you do the test in different populations with different prevalences of the disease. The lower the prevalence, the higher the number of false positives.

Summary box: screening tests

Sensitivity

- Percentage of those with disease who have a positive test result.
- Assessed on patients with 'true' disease: independent of prevalence.
- High sensitivity implies few missed cases and few cases of 'false reassurance'.

Specificity

- Percentage of those without the disease who have a normal test result.
- Assessed on 'truly' normal subjects: independent of disease prevalence.
- High specificity implies few false alarms.

Positive predictive value

- Proportion of those who test positive who truly have the disease. This depends on disease prevalence.
- Useful guide to the balance between true positives and false positives.

TEST YOURSELF: SCREENING

SCREENING and DIAGNOSTIC TESTS

A consultant ophthalmologist with a portable microscope visits the diabetic clinic based at a large group practice and checks the eyes of every patient presenting over several months. The consultant's assessment of whether diabetic retinopathy is present is regarded as the gold standard and his findings are recorded independently of the fundoscopy findings of the single GP running the clinic.

When the results are published, the following statement is made: 'GP fundoscopy; sensitivity 50%, specificity 90%'.

Question

How do you interpret these results?

Suggested answer

The sensitivity of 50% means that the GP is missing half of the cases of diabetic retinopathy identified by the consultant. As this is a primary care clinic, the prevalence of retinopathy is likely to be lower than in a hospital clinic, so a few missed cases will have a significant impact on the numbers correctly identified in practice.

Further analysis would be helpful, because if the GP is missing cases of mild background retinopathy, it may not matter, but if the GP is missing cases of sight-threatening retinopathy, the implications are serious. Further training for the GP (and then reassessment) or a new method of screening might be needed.

The specificity of 90% implies that the GP is correctly identifying 90% of those without retinopathy. A few patients might have simple drusen at the macula which the GP has recorded as diabetic hard exudates. Most GPs would be pleased to get it right so often and would not have a problem with misdiagnosed drusen. But the hospital consultant might point out that there are many more 'normals' than abnormals in the primary care setting and only a small increase in the proportion of such false positives could cause havoc in the clinic if they were all referred for further assessment. Note that the lower the specificity, the higher the proportion of false positives.

SCREENING STATISTICS

Question

What are the (i) sensitivity, (ii) specificity and (iii) positive predictive value in Table 7.3 (Taken from the pneumatic otoscopy example.)?

Table 7.3 Symptomatic children

	Tympanometry positive	Tympanometry negative	Total
Pneumatic positive	150	80	230
Pneumatic negative	50	720	770
Total	200	800	1000

Answers

(i)   The sensitivity (150/200) = 75%
(ii)   The specificity (720/800) = 90%
(iii) The positive predictive value (150/230) = 65%

GLAUCOMA SCREENING IN PRIMARY CARE

Question

Read the following, adapted from Sheldrick and Sharp (1994). Spot six critical points concerning the usefulness and validity of this abstract in reaching the conclusion that general practitioners should screen for glaucoma.

SUMMARY

Background: Previous studies have shown that for every known case of glaucoma there is another case of occult disease. Most cases of glaucoma are detected by optometrists.

Aim: This study set out to determine the prevalence of occult glaucoma in a practice population and assess the likely resource implications of introducing a glaucoma screening programme into a general practice setting.

Method: The 1153 patients registered with one practice in Leicester who were aged 55–69 years on 1 January 1992 and who were not known to have glaucoma prior to screening were invited to a screening clinic. Prior to screening there were 11 known cases of glaucoma in the age group. Screening was carried out by a practice nurse. Patients who failed the screening tests were referred according to the study protocol to the ophthalmology department of the Leicester Royal Infirmary and examined by one ophthalmologist. The number of cases of occult glaucoma and other eye disease detected, the cost per case screened and case detected, and the number of referrals generated were evaluated.

Results: Nine hundred and fifty people (82%) accepted the invitation and attended for glaucoma screening. Of those screened 115 (12%) were referred for ophthalmic assessment. Glaucoma was confirmed in 14 of the referred patients (12%) while a further 15 (13%) were found to have ocular hypertension. All but one of those people diagnosed as having glaucoma recalled having been examined by their optician within the last 5 years; for 50% the period was less than 2 years. Nineteen of the patients referred (17%) had other ocular pathology detected by the ophthalmologist and no abnormality was detected in 65 patients referred (57%). The estimated cost to the practice (excluding hospital outpatient costs) per case screened using the study protocol was £6 and the cost per case detected was £408.

Conclusion: Glaucoma screening may be successfully under-taken in a general practice setting by non-ophthalmically trained staff who have received tuition in the use of the equipment. It is well received by the population served but the capital cost of equipment is likely to be too high for most practices to afford. The reaffirmation of at least one occult case of glaucoma for every known case is particularly alarming in the absence of a national screening programme and the asympto-matic course of this treatable, blinding disease. Closer coop-eration between general practitioners and optometrists will be the practical way ahead for most practices.

Suggested answers

1 Draw the 2×2 table.

		Disease		
		Yes	No	
Test	Positive	29*	86	115
	Negative	?	?	835
		?	?	950

* This figure is 29 if disease is taken to include ocular hypertension.

The negatives were not sent to the consultant and so no gold standard judgement is available to state whether any of them had disease undetected by the screening test. So sensitivity, specificity and negative predictive value of the test cannot be calculated from this study.

The only statistic which can be calculated is the positive predictive value, which is 29/115 (25.2%). Although low, this figure might be perfectly acceptable with its high level of false positives, if costs, anxiety until the consultant diagnosis, and the number of false negatives are all considered to be within reasonable bounds. The 86 false positives represent a price of the screening programme to be balanced against the identification of 29 true positives.

2 The reader cannot tell exactly what screening has achieved. It is possible (although unlikely) that the ophthalmologist would have identified 12% of those screened negative as having glaucoma if they had all been seen by him or her as well. This could be judged if we knew the sensitivity.

3 The screening test was performed in the setting to which it is to be generalized (primary care) and so the value for the positive predictive value is likely to be a reliable estimate for this population. However the validity of the data needs to be known – is the ophthalmologist more likely to diagnose glaucoma in a research setting than in a service programme for example?

4 The 17% with 'other ocular pathology' is an attractive-looking red herring. There might also be 17% of the screened negative population who would have such pathology when examined by the consultant: is there any evidence that the glaucoma screening test is more likely to pick up these other problems? More important, is there any benefit to the patient in identifying this pathology anyway (treatment, palliation, benefit payments etc)? If there is benefit, then a separate study would have to establish the best method to screen for it.

5 It is not clear whether the high proportion of patients who had previously seen the optician was a plus or minus for screening.

   a It is possible that most patients in this age-group (screen positive or screen negative) see an optician over a 5-year period anyway.

   b The optician might be a better investment than GP-based screening.

   c Alternatively it might indicate that re-screening needs to be relatively frequent if the current positives had actually had a negative test at their earlier visit to the optician.

6 It is unusual to exclude hospital outpatient visits from the cost analysis, especially when the number of false positives is high – these might be the most costly part of the exercise.

REFERENCES

de Melker, R.A. (1993) Evaluation of the diagnostic value of pneumatic otoscopy in primary care using the results of typanometry as a reference standard. *British Journal of General Practice*, **43**, 22–4.

Mant, D., and Fowler, G. (1990) Mass screening: theory and ethics. *British Medical Journal*, **300**, 916–8.

Sackett, D.L., Haynes, B.R., Tugwell, P., and Guyatt, G. (1991) *Clinical Epidemiology. A basic science for clinical medicine.* 2nd Edn. Boston: Little, Brown and Co.

Sheldrick, J.H., and Sharp, A. (1994) Glaucoma screening clinic in general practice: prevalence of occult disease, and resource implications. *British Journal of General Practice*, **44**, 561–5.

Wiggelinkhuizen, J., Maytham D., and Hanslo, D. (1988) Dipstick screening for urinary tract infection. *South African Medical Journal*, **74**, 224–8.

Wilson, J.M.G. (1976) Some principles of early diagnosis and detection. In: *Proceedings of a colloquium, Magdalen College, Oxford*. Ed. G. Teeling-Smith. Office of Health Economics.

Woodward, M.N., and Griffiths, D.M. (1993) Use of dipsticks for routine analysis of urine from children with acute abdominal pain. *British Medical Journal*, **306**, 1512.

8

Other types of evidence

We have focused on traditional study methodology, which has its roots in mathematics, logic and clinical epidemiology. This chapter simply draws attention to other methods which may be of equal or greater relevance to research projects in primary care, but does not attempt to detail the role of critical reading in assessing the output from such studies. Other publications should be consulted, such as Ridsdale (1996).

QUALITATIVE STUDIES

The precision of counts and measurements might seem worlds away from the hurly-burly of daily surgery. How do you gather evidence about ideas, attitudes and feelings, which are not easily summarized or quantified? One answer is to listen, record and observe, without putting numbers or figures to the material. Such qualitative research has been used extensively in the social sciences and there are good texts and reviews, such as Mays and Pope (1996).

'I didn't like to trouble the doctor, like – it's only a bit of rheumatism. Although I must say it does stop me getting up and down stairs like I used to – and I wish I could find someone to walk the dog on days when it is bad'

Quotes like this – the sort of thing a primary care worker may hear every day – can contain important information and perspectives on a research topic. How do you approach it critically?

1 A different sort of representativeness

Do not demand random samples of this sort of data. It is likely that individuals will have been selected as individuals because they represent certain types of patient or certain issues, or because they are in a specific position at work or in their community, which means they represent points of view or feelings which the research wants to draw on.

> 'A group of women were chosen, who were from working class households, with young families, to discuss their attitudes towards the children's diet'
> 'Health needs in the local community were assessed through in-depth interviews with a local councillor, playgroup leader, patients' representative, carer, teacher, parent teachers' association chair'

Unless such a sample is random and large enough for statistical comparison, it is inappropriate to analyse it with the sort of summary statistics outlined in Chapter 4. There are various approaches to analysis – searching for themes, identifying words or phrases or other textual sections, which recur or form a pattern for example. An important feature of this type of research is that the approaches used in any study are made explicit.

2 Theory and ideas are important

Qualitative researchers are not simply regurgitating people's language in a string of quotes. The themes and the drawing out of ideas are designed to develop certain ideas – those ideas fuel the content and style of the interviews. The analysis may then be used to develop specific theories which both explain and are illustrated by the quotes and the extracted themes. There are systematic approaches to this and once again it is characteristic that the underlying theory is clearly elucidated for the reader.

Example

The position adopted in this study is that the people who are its subjects have responses to medicine and what it can offer them which are rational, and their understanding of what is or is not within their power to control as far as their health is concerned is realistic from their own point of view (Cornwell, 1984).

It is the themes and ideas, as well as the populations studied, which have to be put to the test of external validity: are they relevant, what are the implications, and how useful might they be in practice?

Often such research raises issues about awareness, attitudes and education of health professionals and patients, as much as it does about precise interventions and outcomes. For example, Cornwell, in the study quoted from above, analyses the views on general practitioners of the East End families she interviews, and concludes that there are three main points of criticism of doctors: failure to diagnose or making the wrong diagnosis; not making clinical examinations or doing clinical tests; always ending with a prescription or prescribing the same medicine for different conditions.

Reflection stop

- How can studies which report patients' views be incorporated into daily practice – is it that such patients need more understanding of the difficulties and vagueness of diagnostics in general practice?
- How do you square these patients' views on prescribing with qualitative studies on doctors in which doctors feel patients are too demanding of prescriptions?
- Is such a study 'evidence' on which you would feel you might act?

3 Multiple methods can be used to collect data

These range from focus groups to in-depth interviews with individuals, or the use of documentary material.

THE META-ANALYSIS OR SYSTEMATIC OVERVIEW

Those of you who want to do some serious critical reading are urged to read one of a growing number of texts about the 'new science' of systematic reviewing, such as Chalmers and Altman (1995).

The old days of reviewing a topic by selecting some papers, giving them all some space in the review, gently chiding some and praising others, and reaching some sort of overall view on the topic are numbered. Such is the enormous amount of information, the argument goes, that we have the following duties:

1 Track down everything relevant on a particular topic. That may mean identifying unpublished material or material in obscure journals, searching specialist publications by hand, writing to the authors for details not shown in their papers, going outside the academic channels of publication for material (reports from government agencies or drug companies for example). This is the world of the 'systematic search'.
2 Set up explicit criteria by which studies will or will not be considered for the overview. For example, if it is decided that uncontrolled studies are not acceptable, they are simply not included once they have been identified as such.
3 Judge the validity of those studies that remain after your selection criteria have been applied, using the types of principles outlined in the earlier sections of this book (selection bias, information bias, etc). Some authors construct a validity score, although it is not always clear how much weight should be placed on different items. This process can be more or less technical. For example, in reviews of randomized controlled trials, it is common for a study to be marked down if it has not detailed the actual method of randomization – it might have been done perfectly well, but if it has not been clearly stated, the reviewer cannot know this.
4 Work in groups to stay sane. This is the basis of the Cochrane collaboration, groups around the world voluntarily reviewing literature on their chosen topics. There is also a technical aspect to this in that the validity of reviewers' assessments can be checked by comparing results in a formal manner.

TEST YOURSELF: SYSTEMATIC REVIEW OF NECK TREATMENTS

It is not the intention of this text to go further than to indicate that there is a whole science out there on this topic. However, the critical reader might well wish to read and make a judgement on a systematic review. They are increasingly appearing as papers, often in journals such as the *British Medical Journal* and the *British Journal of General Practice.*

Question

Here is an abstract from such a review, taken from Aker (1996). Read the abstract and write a paragraph for your local practice newsletter which summarizes your interpretation of the review in simple terms.

ABSTRACT

Objective: To review the efficacy of conservative management of mechanical neck disorders.

Methods: Published and unpublished reports were identified through computerized and manual searches of bibliographical databases, reference lists from primary articles, and letters to authors, agencies, foundations, and content experts. Selection criteria were applied to blinded articles, and selected articles were scored for methodological quality. Effect sizes were calculated from raw pain scores and combined by using meta-analytic techniques when appropriate.

Results: Twenty-four randomized clinical trials met the selection criteria and were categorized by type of intervention: 9 used manual treatments; 12 physical medicine methods; 4 drug treatment; and 3 education of patients (4 trials investigated more than one form of intervention). The intervention strategies were summarized separately. Pooling of studies was considered only within each category. Five of the nine trials that used manual treatment in combination with other treatments were combined. One to four weeks after treatment the pooled effect size was −0.6 (95% confidence interval −0.9 to −0.4), equivalent to an improvement of 16 (6.9 to 23.1) points on a 100 point scale. Sensitivity analyses on study quality, chronicity, and data imputation did not alter this estimate. For other interventions, studies could not be combined to arrive at pooled estimates of effect.

Conclusions: There is little information available from clinical trials to support many of the treatments for mechanical neck pain. In general, conservative interventions have not been studied in enough detail to assess efficacy or effectiveness adequately.

Note the main points:

1 The focus on the extensiveness of the literature review – it is a specific feature of this type of overview that attempts are made to trace *all* potentially relevant studies.
2 The rigorous selection of studies on the basis of preselected explicit criteria of quality – no longer is it a matter of quoting everything published on a topic in a chatty fashion, it is a business of identifying everything published and then carrying out a standardized selection exercise.
3 Meta-analysis is a statistical procedure to combine the results of different studies – it cannot correct for variations in quality or method, however.
4 'Effect size' is an attempt to estimate the actual effect of an intervention, not simply whether it was 'statistically significant' or not.
5 'Sensitivity analyses' involve techniques in which assumptions about the quality of data are varied to see what effect they might have on the result of the meta-analysis.

Reflection stop

Regrettably the conclusion of the abstract is a common one, seen at the end of many a rigorous overview – there is insufficient good evidence to form a scientific judgement on efficacy.

How do you interpret this in your own approach to neck pain treatment?

Does NO evidence mean NO action? Does the small improvement noted mean 'Well, at least, it does no harm, so carry on with your particular favourite'?

Would you share the result with your patients?

The problem is that absence of evidence does not mean that there is active evidence against doing such treatments. If you decide to use manual treatments, the overview is simply saying that you are not acting on available scientific evidence – but neither are you acting against it. It simply ain't there – and so belief, experience, patient wishes, your gut feeling and all such alternative evidence must come into play.

REFERENCES

Aker, P.D., Gross, A.R., Goldsmith, C.H., and Peloso, P. (1996) Conservative management of mechanical neck pain: systematic overview and meta-analysis. *British Medical Journal*, **313**, 1291–6.

Chalmers, I., and Altman, D.G. (1995) *Systematic reviews*. BMJ Publishing Group.

Cornwell, J. (1984) *Hard-earned lives. Accounts of health and illness from East London*. Tavistock Publications.

Mays, N., and Pope, C. (1996) *Qualitative research in health care*. BMJ Books.

Ridsdale, L. (1995) *Evidence-based general practice. A critical reader*. London: W.B. Saunders Co.

9

Tackling the tabloids

So is this critical reading stuff of any use other than helping to pass the Membership of the Royal College of General Practitioners and providing an alternative to the lunchtime talk as a route to postgraduate educational points and allowances?

We think so because we believe that for some of you it will brighten up practice and make clinical work potentially more effective. But we also think so because the need for a critical perspective is not restricted to the rather dry world of reading the medical literature.

This section is about critical reading outside the medical scientific journals: the Monday morning syndrome of the patient with the rolled-up *Sunday Times*, ready to flatten you with the latest medical revelation; the drug rep with the flip chart of extraordinarily convincing barcharts; the patient with a photocopy of a magical diet taken from a recent book; and increasingly there is the Internet.

How do you cope? The principles are the same as for the scientific literature. Here are some examples.

1 **'Men are 80% more likely to get backache when they are married'**

A headline from a newspaper report of a conference where cross-sectional data had been presented showing that married men were more likely to get backache than single men. There was an odds ratio of 1.8 for the association (which is 80% higher than the reference odds of 1.0 – hence the headline).

Points to hang on to:

a Odds are not the same as risks. When you have something common like back pain the odds ratio can be a distorted estimate of the increased risk – it will tend to be an overestimate. So an odds ratio of 1.8 for the association between marital status and back pain cannot simply be translated as 'married men have an 80% higher risk'.

b When given a relative term ('80% higher than . . .'), ask for absolute terms – what is the actual risk of back pain in men, and what might the extra risk actually be in married men. A small risk multiplied by 1.8 will still be a small risk; a big risk multiplied by 1.8 might become a huge risk.

c In cross-sectional studies particularly, association does not imply cause. It may be that the type of men who get married are more likely to have an already established back pain pattern. A different headline might have read 'back pain sufferers are at higher risk of getting married'.

2 **'Women on third generation oral contraceptive pills are twice as likely to have a deep venous thrombosis (DVT) than women on first or second generation pills'**

Once again think absolute and be wary of relative terms ('twice as likely'). For the individual woman, the important question is the actual risk of DVT and what 'twice as likely' means in actual risk terms (i.e. what extra risk of DVT can be attributed to the third generation pills?).

Here are some figures taken from Guillebaud (1995):

- incidence of DVT in non-users of the pill: 7 per 100 000 women per year;
- incidence of DVT in users of 1st/2nd generation pills: 15 per 100 000 women per year;
- incidence of DVT in users of 3rd generation pills: 30 per 100 000 women per year;
- incidence of DVT during pregnancy: 90 per 100 000 women per year.

The doubling of risk from old to new generation pills actually means an extra 15 cases of DVT per year among every 100 000 users of third generation pills. This can be compared with an extra 83 cases among 100 000 pregnant women over the base-line risk in non-pregnant women who are not using the oral contraceptive.

3 'Liver cancer link to the pill'

This is another variation on the absolute risk theme. Links between unusual events and common exposures appear often in the epidemiological literature: overhead electricity and childhood cancer, VDU operation and spontaneous abortions. How do we interpret this for our patients?

First such studies are not to be derided. They may play an important part in policy making. The large investment in investigating links between cancer and nuclear power installations is crucial. If nuclear power carries a small but definite risk of leukaemia for example, it raises important questions about the expansion of nuclear power: a small risk spread wide will cause a significant number of cases.

But in primary care it is the worried individual rather than issues of policy making which is the concern. One simple way of dealing with this is to ask two questions:

a Given that a child has cancer, what is the risk that they may live near electricity pylons? This expresses the need to know what proportion of all childhood cancers might be caused by living near electricity pylons. It is likely to be small.

b Given that a child lives near an electricity pylon, what is the risk that they will develop childhood cancer? This will be small, even if it is a little higher than for children who do not live near an electricity pylon.

This sort of reasoning does not give an answer to 'should I move house?' but it does give some sense of individual risk as against the published observation of a 'link'.

So what about the oral contraceptive pill and liver cancer? In Britain liver cancer in young women is exceedingly rare. However, a significant proportion of the cases have been attributed to the pill, since most of the very few young women who do develop liver cancer have used the pill. Yet so rare is the cancer, that the risk of any woman on the pill developing it is exceedingly small. This is an instance where the paper is technically right (there is a link) but where there is little basis for a 'scare' around individual risk.

4 'Our drug has been subjected to rigorous randomized controlled trials'

This is usually true of any new drug nowadays. The sophistication of trials in clinical practice means that drug companies are often at the forefront of methods and study design, and good trials are done. Using our jargon, internal validity is often strong.

The catch is that the internal validity is used to steamroller the use of a drug, when it is external validity which needs close inspection. The question to put to the drug rep is 'who took part in the trials?'. A typical selection of primary care patients or highly selected hospital patients or volunteers? Drug trials in heart failure or osteoarthritis, for example, are in practice going to be prescribed overwhelmingly for older people: were the studies done on this group? People who agree to take part and who are included in trials are often very different from those patients who are eligible for treatment in everyday practice.

5 'The gene for osteoporosis has been identified. Professor Ben Density said that this could mean young girls being screened for the condition which is responsible for many hip fractures among elderly women'

This is a caricature of the torrent of press releases which accompany the hunt for the genes of human disease. It begs many questions.

The identification of a gene in most cases will mean that a genetic marker has been found to be increased in frequency in patients with the particular disease. In other words there is an association between the marker and the disease. As we learned in the screening section of the book, this does not answer the question of how many women would be correctly classified by this gene as likely to develop osteoporosis: what would the predictive values be if the test were applied in the community?

Also important is the question of the use to which such a test would be put, even if it did correctly classify a young girl's future osteoporotic career. What preventive approaches are available? If the answer were to encourage exercise in those at risk, why not encourage exercise in all young women rather than identify individuals with the message that you might be at higher risk of a hip fracture in 60 years? What are the social and psychological implications of imparting such knowledge to the genetically disadvantaged?

6 'At the lunchtime meeting Ms Angiogram, the new vascular surgeon, encouraged the GPs to send all their transient ischaemic attacks (TIAs) to her'

This is a common statement, usually landing on cynical ears of GPs used to long waiting lists and wondering why the surgeons want to make them longer.

Does the surgeon know what she is saying? What she means is: 'send me neat, clearcut, clinically probable TIAs like I am used to seeing and investigating in outpatients'. Out there in the dirty world of real consulters, there are dizzy do's and odd symptoms in regular presenters, which form a messy ragbag of 'possible TIAs'. Send them all up and the response might be: poor diagnostic acumen by the GP, why are they sending me these trivial problems?

But let us suppose that a protocol is agreed and GPs put it into practice efficiently and send up all the probables. The reason for the surgeon's encouragement is that she can arrange instant duplex scanning of the carotid arteries and she has presented convincing randomized controlled trial evidence that carotid artery surgery is beneficial. End of story?

Well, no. With your critical reader's hat on, you want to know how many positive scans will there be? (Answer: quite a lot.) How many of those do the trials clearly show would benefit from surgery? (Answer: a minority.) Have you the resources to do surgery if you do scan them all? (Answer: yes, if you are paying.)

Once again, some simple questions based on the logic of screening and on the external validity of trial evidence can put dogmatic statements (albeit ones from which much positive help can be gleaned) into some sort of context.

7 'I've read about this diet, doctor. Do you think it will help my rheumatism?'

The range of responses to this in surgeries up and down the land must be vast, and will reflect the personality, psychology and interests of the doctor and patient, as much as anything else. Has critical reading anything to offer?

Let us suppose for a moment that you want to spend time sorting out an answer. The first step might be to look in the literature to see if there has been a systematic review of trials of the efficacy of diet in rheumatic complaints – or more than one review. If there has not been such an overview, you could consider doing one yourself, although this is a big undertaking nowadays with its own methods of investigation, collaboration and funding. If this gives a clearcut answer, this can be used as part of the discussion with the patient.

The problem with so many of the problems which are uncertain treatment areas is that the conclusion of any overview is likely to be 'there are not enough good studies' and 'there is no convincing evidence of efficacy'. This need not be entirely negative: the point can be shared with the patient that 'science simply does not know'. You can move on to discuss other reasons for using or not using the diet. What is important for the critical reader is that 'lack of evidence' or 'no strong evidence for an effect' should not be translated into 'strong evidence against'. This is a prescription for nihilism, since much of what we do in general practice still does not possess randomized trial evidence for or against.

Reflection stop

- Think absolutes if given a 'relative' statement.
- Think predictive values and usefulness if given open access to a screening, diagnostic or treatment service.
- Think external validity especially if given a trial result.
- Lack of evidence does not mean 'don't do it'.

TEST YOURSELF: BONE DENSITY SCREENING – TO BUY OR NOT TO BUY?

A patient comes in to see you who has read in the local newspaper that the District Health Authority is refusing to buy a bone densitometer to screen the local female population because there is 'no evidence' that it is beneficial. The article said also that some general practices are thinking of clubbing together to buy their own. 'It's scandalous that we may be going around with this bone disease and not knowing about it. Are you going to buy into the service, doctor?'

Question

What information would you like to have in order to answer this question?

Suggested answer

1 The Health Authority were talking about screening the female population as a whole. You would like to know whether such screening of the 'fit and well' would be advantageous – is there evidence that the local population as a whole would benefit? There are a number of hidden implications of screening that always need to be clarified – essentially it is all about Wilson's criteria again (see page 163) – notably how good is the test at selecting those who will benefit from treatment and how good is the treatment? If HRT is the assumed treatment, is there a clear policy on dosage and duration of treatment? What are the side-effects, given that it is well women who are being screened? What is known about compliance and would it be good enough to justify a population screening programme?

2 What the newspaper and the questioner may be confusing is an individual's desire to be investigated and treated and the trickier question of whether a population programme to actively encourage screening is justified. There may be, for example, a far more cogent argument for a densitometry service if it is to be used to diagnose osteoporosis in women at high risk, for example those on long-term steroid treatment. Even here you would wish to know that bone densitometry is reliable, will contribute to the decision on how to manage the individual patient, and that treatment is available and effective in those at high risk.

The point that the newspapers may ignore is that the simple availability of a screening test does not mean that a screening programme is a useful or beneficial thing. More evidence is needed!

CONCLUDING THOUGHTS TO THE FIRST PART OF THE BOOK

Reflection, not evangelism

Our message is simple. The most important skill in practical critical reading is the logical thinking through of the implications and consequences of putting the result into practice. Often the authors have not done this – indeed they often cannot do it, in the sense that they cannot know or cater for the particular context in which each reader works.

So reflective reading is an active and crucial part of the scientific endeavour – the willingness of health workers to engage their common sense and their experience in a dialogue with the study results, and tackle the all-important issue of 'what would happen if . . .'.

Sure, develop the skills to appraise the science of the studies if you wish – and some of this book is about that. But the evangelists have encouraged a misconception – that critical reading means we all have to do our own systematic review of every topic before deciding whether the study is good or not. Well, even if that were your inclination, timetabling alone ridicules this.

Much more important, as a *general* skill, is the equally intellectually demanding process of reflective thinking about the implications of the study – not a bundle of esoteric mathematical skills, but logic and experience and some lateral thinking.

Happy reflections!

REFERENCES

Guillebaud, J. (1995) Advising women on which pill to take. *British Medical Journal*, **311**, 1111–2.

Part II

Critical reading and reflective practice

10

Paralysed by the literature?

READING ABOUT TOPICS

In the first section of this book, we have been concerned with the analysis of individual publications. Now it is time to consider a different sort of approach where a topic is the starting point rather than a specific paper. For many working in primary care, this seems appropriate because questions about improving quality are usually generated by individual cases or problems rather than by the spontaneous reading of an article in a journal. This is sometimes referred to as problem-based learning and has been shown to be a highly effective method of keeping up-to-date. Even after several years in practice it is possible to master the skills involved, for example by participating in case-based journal clubs (Sackett and Haynes, 1995). Events in clinical practice are analysed with the aim of defining a problem or problems to which the literature may help provide some solutions. Reflection on practice is the starting point.

REFLECTING ON YOUR WORKING KNOWLEDGE

We will assume that the reader is faced, like the authors, with a number of obvious problems and uncertainties in primary care and is not in a position to have to go looking for more. One aim of this section of the book is to empower you to use your own knowledge and experience in this way. For this reason, in the chapters which follow, we will ask you to pause and reflect on your own working knowledge in order to identify your own agenda for reading the literature.

The process of reflecting on practice and modifying and restructuring our understanding in the face of uncertainty or surprise has been described as an essential component of a professional's activity (Schon, 1983). In *The Reflective Practitioner*, Schon also postulates that:

> '...as practice becomes more repetitive and routine ... the practitioner may miss important opportunities to think about what he is doing ... And if he learns, as often happens, to be selectively inattentive to phenomena that do not fit the categories of his knowing-in-action, then he may suffer from boredom or "burnout" and afflict his clients with the consequences of his narrowness and rigidity.'

Schon's concept of knowing-in-action is a way of describing the tacit knowledge which informs practice. The process of reflection on and modification of such knowledge is central to professional practice and could be seen as the **art** of critical reading which complements the science of critical reading and the use of the skills of critical appraisal. Reflection on current practice is the most powerful starting point.

An overview of the process leading from reflection to a change in practice is given in Figure 10.1 which summarizes the themes of this chapter. Note that sometimes general curiosity will drive a literature search, but that when the search process is problem-based, the questions generated are usually more specific and the potential for learning and improving professional performance is greater. So we will begin by discussing one form of reflection: critical incident analysis.

Critical incident analysis

Sometimes terms such as 'significant event auditing' or 'critical incident analysis' are used to describe a particular approach to problem-based learning (Pietroni and Millard, 1996). Reflection on practice leads to the identification of an important event which has the potential to stimulate learning both from the experience and

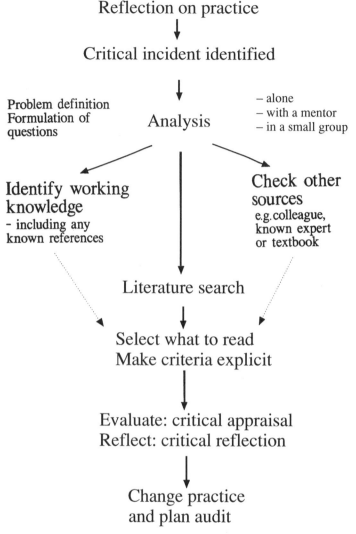

Figure 10.1 Overview of the process leading from reflection to change in practice.

from the literature and most importantly from the interaction between the two.

Critical incident analysis involves analysis of a critical incident which is 'over and above the routine', which can 'trouble, exasperate or frustrate us' or which provides an 'example of effective or ineffective practice' (O'Dowd, 1993). The incident does not have to be clinical; a non-clinical example would be analysis of a patient who leaves the practice but does not change address (O'Dowd, 1993). What is crucial is that the analysis focuses on a particular area of interest unlike, for example, random case analysis. It is also important that those involved give an account of what has actually happened rather than rely on generalizations or opinions (Bradley, 1996).

The analysis is systematic – aiming to identify events or behaviours which have been critical (beneficial or detrimental) to the outcome. The analysis is based on the factual account of the event and aims to minimize the effects of subjective opinion, generalization and personal judgement. In order to do this it is necessary to have a description in which the specific reasons for actions are clear and obvious without the need for interpretation based on a pre-existing theory (Bradley, 1996).

In facilitated case discussion in a small group context, the facilitator may use specific techniques for making group analysis of critical incidents 'safe' and effective (Robinson *et al.*, 1995). These may be similar to those of Pendleton who summarized a set of rules for analysing videotapes of consultations (Pendleton *et al.*, 1984). These are summarized in Box 10.1.

Box 10.1 Pendleton's rules for analysing videotapes of consultations (after Pendleton *et al.*, 1984).

1 Brief factual statement, then watch video.
2 You speak first and comment on strengths.
3 Group adds comments on strengths.
4 Group makes recommendations (not criticisms).
5 Summary by group leader of strengths and recommendations.
6 Role play of recommendations.

An alternative approach emphasizes the importance of the practitioner explicitly asking the group for help and stating what he or she was hoping to achieve in the consultation (Silverman, Kurtz and Draper, 1996). This approach is summarized in Figure 10.2.

The Calgary Cambridge Approach to Consulation Analysis
(Based on Silverman *et al.*,1996): mnemonic ASDA

A   Ask the group for help

Pendleton's rules seem to emphazise ever-present
danger in their insistence on rigid ordering of feedback
and may prevent the practitioner from saying what her
learning needs are. Here safety is ensured by the
facilitator making sure that an explicit 'ask the group
for help' statement is made once the video has been
seen. This is the crucial thing in making it safe because
few people are destructive when their help is solicited.

S   Specify the desired outcome

Under Pendleton, comments are made which are
often judgemental: 'that was a good consultation' or
'first talk about the good things'. Here the emphasis is
on what the doctor is hoping to achieve and making this
explicit. Then interventions are only more or less
successful in terms of the desired outcome. This is another
way of making the whole process less judgmental and
therefore less threatening.

D   Describe accurately what occurs and the consequences

Once the tape has been seen and the practitioner
has identified the problem area, part of the tape may
be reviewed so that everyone can note accurately
what happened. Interpretation from the group should
be minimal but the consequences of interventions can
be reflected to the practitioner for his comments.

A   Act out alternative suggestions

The practitioner should then be encouraged to develop
suggestions for alternative approaches and these should
then be rehearsed using role play. Adults learn through
'doing' and role play here is not an 'added extra' or
an 'optional extra' as it sometimes seems in Pendleton,
but the goal towards which the group work is moving.

Figure 10.2 Alternative approach: the importance of the practitioner
stating aims of consultation.

In order to 'turn anecdote into data', it is necessary to reduce the effect of subjectivity and hence the analysis should ideally include more than one person (Bradley, 1996). In the context of learning, Pietroni describes critical event analysis between just two doctors who are co-mentoring (Pietroni and Millard, 1996). A number of techniques may be used in the process of analysis, including brainstorming and role play as well as more traditional small group discussion (Minghella and Benson, 1995). However, Havelock and Schofield have pointed out that opportunities for working in groups to discuss cases are most readily available for GP registrars and trainers, leaving the majority of primary care practitioners relatively isolated (Havelock and Schofield, 1996).

In its loosest sense, critical incident analysis could refer to an individual reflecting alone about a significant event of relevance to practice. The point is that the whole process is far more creative, more effective and less open to collusion if an external resource is used to illuminate what has happened and facilitate reflection (Robinson *et al.*, 1995). One of the external resources to which even the most isolated practitioner may have access is the published literature.

Once an analysis of a specific incident has occurred, the next step is to check other incidents for similarities and differences in order to refine the conclusions which have been drawn. Balint emphasized both the potential of every consultation for analysis and also the individuality of each case. This may have distracted practitioners from the need to concentrate on particular critical incidents and from the potential of aggregating cases to find a common pattern (O'Dowd, 1993). O'Dowd has this to say:

'Can the cases we discuss be linked together into a series? . . . Instead of Mrs Jones with the bad back, can we reframe the problem into "backs that won't get better". Instead of Mr Smith who always wants referral, is it possible to measure the number of patient initiated referrals in the practice and then deal with any questions arising from such a measurement. This can be a natural progression from critical incident analysis. The observation of one critical incident may reverberate in the experience of members of the primary care team, and by exciting their interest and imagination may encourage them to report similar cases so that a pattern may develop.'

It is often at this stage, when several incidents with a common theme have occurred, that an individual or a group make the decision to search the literature. Because critical incident analysis is inductive, aiming to describe key skills or behaviours without reference to pre-existing theory, it may be particularly useful in three contexts:

1 education, both for learning, curriculum development and assessment;
2 audit where the behaviours under scrutiny are used to generate standards and as a basis for change;
3 in qualitative research to identify important elements in a complex process such as decision-making about diagnostic tests, prescribing or referral (Bradley, 1992).

Here the analysis is being used to generate specific questions based on real problems with the aim of improving professional performance; hence the first two categories apply.

Before searching the literature, it is important to identify what you already know about the problem or topic. Thinking laterally and broadly about all aspects which may be relevant enables the specific problem identified to be seen in context. Discussion with others will help to identify 'what else you need to know'.

FORMULATING AN ANSWERABLE QUESTION

Sackett, Richardson and Haynes (1997) have emphasized the importance of the process which leads from a problem in practice to the formulation of an answerable question. They concentrate on the areas to which evidence-based medicine may be able to provide answers, very often in a quantitative way. The first stage is discovering 'a specific decision or action that you don't know enough about to tackle confidently'. This is called a 'knowledge gap'. The next stage is to ask a question which is 'well built, by which we mean both directly relevant to patients' problems and phrased in ways that direct your search to relevant and precise answers' (Sackett, Richardson and Haynes, 1997). Four components of a well-built question are identified and these are summarized in Box 10.2.

Box 10.2 Four components of a well-built question (Sackett *et al.*, 1997; with permission).

1 The patient or problem being addressed.
2 The intervention being considered, whether by nature or by clinical design (a cause, a prognostic factor, a treatment, etc).
3 A comparison intervention, when relevant.
4 The clinical outcome or outcomes of interest.

Approaching the literature

So how do we now go to the literature to find out about a topic or to answer a specific question generated in clinical practice, rather than starting with an individual paper?

A number of starting points are summarized below:

- a specific question identified after critical incident analysis;
- a memory of reading a paper on a topic which you want to find;
- a paper suggested by an expert you have asked;
- a paper described or quoted in a textbook;
- a search for 'secondary references' quoted in papers you have already read;
- a desire to review the literature of the topic you are interested in without a specific author or reference in mind.

The problem is that the literature often seems daunting and vast. Occasionally a single crucial paper can be identified which may help to solve the problem, in which case the skills developed in the first part of this book will be valuable in assessing the implications for primary care. More often, however, the published literature will include a large number of papers, each with a slightly different view of the subject and sometimes reaching apparently different conclusions.

It is easy to feel paralysed by the sheer amount of weighty knowledge there is to acquire. It can all seem overwhelming and it may seem impossible to know where to start. Often you will use a combination of different starting points. The end result should be a small pile of references (or at least titles or abstracts), and it is important to acknowledge that however careful the search, there is always an element of luck in what you find.

Getting started

If you have difficulty getting started, there are several strategies for overcoming 'reader's block'. Basing your reading on a real problem is the most obvious. There are a number of other tips which can help if you have got stuck. These are summarized in Box 10.3 and discussed below.

Box 10.3 How to overcome reader's block.

- Work with colleagues.
- Start with an easy topic.
- Start with a superficial approach.
- Get help from a medical librarian.
- Learn how to use Medline yourself.
- Don't try to cram.

Work with colleagues

Working in small groups with colleagues is usually a mutually sustaining process in thinking and reading about a topic. Tasks can be divided up and shared and ideas developed by the group. Remember that a group can be more productive than the sum of the performances of each individual.

Start with an easy topic

It helps to start with a relatively well-defined topic where there are only a few key papers to read and summarize. Once you have successfully tackled such a subject, even if only superficially, the block to getting started will have been broken down.

Start with a superficial approach

Try not to be too obsessional about reading absolutely everything about a topic. If you begin with a conscious decision to be rather superficial, you will at least be able to make a start and you will obtain an overview of the topic. You may then make an informed choice about how to use the remaining time for checking particular areas in greater depth.

Jewell and Freeman describe three levels of reading in Jones and Kinmonth (1995) and these are summarized in Box 10.4.

Box 10.4 Three levels of reading. From Jewell and Freeman in Jones and Kinmonth (1995) with permission.

1 **Browsing**; 'everyday material that happens to cross one's path'.
2 **Reading for information**; to answer 'questions concerning individual patient's problems . . . audit, and the care and management of the whole practice'.
3 **Reading for research**; 'demands a more systematic approach to the search'.

Greenhalgh points out that both information and pleasure are derived from browsing and that overdoing critical appraisal risks killing the enjoyment of casual reading (Greenhalgh, 1997). The main focus here is on the second category: reading for information. This is sometimes used to answer a very specific question generated by a clinical encounter, but often is simply to get general information quickly about a well-defined topic. 'We don't have a particular paper in mind or a very specific question to ask and we aren't aiming for an exhaustive overview of the literature. We just want to know, say, what's the latest expert advice on drug treatment of asthma or whether anything new has been written on whooping cough vaccine' (Greenhalgh, 1997). So you don't need to be too obsessional about finding every single paper (as you might if you were reading for research) and it is perfectly reasonable to start by being only just a little more purposive than browsing by asking some fairly general questions.

Get help from a medical librarian

Enlist the help of your nearest medical librarian and if possible learn how to use the new technology for searching and scanning abstracts of papers. It is particularly important to get some hands-on tuition with computerized systems like 'Medline'. These are available in most postgraduate centre libraries or by modem link to the British Medical Association or via the Internet.

There is a steep learning curve: a small amount of supervised teaching will increase your effectiveness greatly and save considerable time. It is also worth remembering that however impressive the technology, it may still be worthwhile doing a manual search. The indexing of computerized databases can be quite limited in their present form and it is well worth pursuing references quoted by others.

Learn how to use Medline yourself

A number of different electronic databases are available. Medline is probably the most commonly used by those in primary care because of its breadth of coverage, its currency (frequently updated) and the flexibility of search options. This breadth and flexibility is a two-edged sword because it is also large and complex. Most searches take 10–30 minutes to perform, so it is unlikely that many clinicians will incorporate its use into routine consultations with patients. However, attempts are being made to deliver evidence in an accessible form in the consultation and this is generally referred to as 'clinical decision support'. How this may add value to the consultation has been summarized (Baker, Maskrey and Kirk, 1997) in Figure 10.3 and is reproduced from Baker *et al.* with permission.

In her book *How to Read a Paper*, Trisha Greenhalgh devotes her longest chapter to searching the literature using Medline and this excellent introduction should be compulsory reading for the novice (Greenhalgh, 1997). Here we will merely highlight a few important concepts. Firstly, 'If you are computerless, make friends with a librarian; if you are computer phobic, sign up for desensitization right away!' (Sackett, Richardson and Haynes, 1997).

Secondly, remember that there are two main ways of searching on a subject, using either the indexed headings of the database or by using free text words which might appear in the title or abstract of papers. The former are called **MeSH**: medical subject headings defined by the National Library of Medicine of the United States; spelling is in American English and can sometimes create problems. Usually, when you type your subject into the computer, it spends 15 seconds 'mapping to medical subject headings' and allows you to

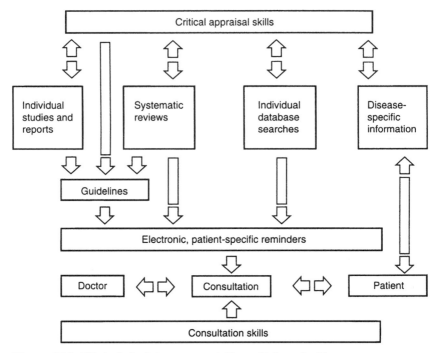

Figure 10.3 Clinical decision support (from Baker et al.)

choose the most appropriate ones. This hierarchical system is the core structure of the database, so a basic understanding helps. Learn how to find your way around this thesaurus. In particular, learn how to 'explode' a heading to generate its subheadings and how these can be used to broaden or narrow the focus of a search. The alternative way of searching is to use **textwords** (tw). This method is most useful for concepts which are not systematically indexed or for jargon terms not recognized by the indexers; for example, 'heartsink patients'. Textwords can also be useful as a methodological filter when only a particular design of study is felt to be relevant; for example, adding terms such as 'risk', 'odds ratio' or 'sensitivity' which are not systematically indexed at present.

Thirdly, remember the aim is to start broad so that important papers aren't missed, but then to focus down and narrow the search so that only relevant articles are selected. The simple ways in which sets from within the database are combined in this way are referred to by the daunting term '**Boolean operators**'. These refer to the search strategy terms 'or', 'and' and 'not'. Using 'or' broadens a search by simply combining sets together whereas 'and' restricts the focus to articles in common between the different sets. 'Not' also refines a search, narrowing the focus by excluding certain terms.

Finally, you need to be aware of the different ways in which you can limit a search. For example, there are options to restrict to English language papers only or to journals held in your local library ('local holdings'). When searching using MeSH terms, you have the option to 'restrict to focus'; that is confine your search to articles where the search term is a major theme rather than just mentioned in discussion. Particularly useful for answering specific evidence-based medicine questions are the limiters based on study methodology. For example, publication type (pt) restrictions include review article, controlled trial, meta-analysis and practice guideline, to name but a few.

The contribution of these concepts to a search strategy are summarized in Figure 10.4 which is based on the approach to teaching used by Sackett, Richardson and Haynes (1997). These concepts are hard to grasp without practical examples. If you are unfamiliar with them, it may be helpful to use the diagram as a syllabus for working on your own (e.g. with the examples given by Greenhalgh referred to above) or to help formulate areas for supervised training.

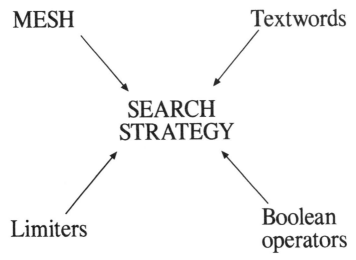

Figure 10.4 Four components of a search strategy, based on Sackett, Richardson and Haynes (1997).

Don't try to cram

You will gain little if you attempt to cram your brain with weighty evidence. A few key ideas are easier to assimilate, to remember and to discuss, and if your search has been stimulated by a real problem, they might even influence the way you practice.

Selecting what to read

The next stage involves selecting the most appropriate articles to read by a quick evaluation of the title and abstract, asking whether if the conclusions are correct, you will be affected by the results (Jones and Kinmonth, 1995). Articles may be of interest for many different reasons and sometimes there will be a strong element of personal choice in the selection. Nevertheless, it is worth trying to be clear as to why you are including a specific article because this is the first critical part of the process. We like to classify the main reasons for reading an article into a number of simple categories (Box 10.5).

Box 10.5 Reasons for selecting an article to read.

- Interesting title.
- Findings potentially useful.
- Apparent influence of paper (e.g. often quoted by others, 'citation index').
- Knowledge of authors, e.g. having previously read something good by same author.
- An exciting or new idea.
- Availability of journal and its familiarity.

Of course there may well be other reasons for reading an article and sometimes there will be overlap between categories. The important point is to make a conscious effort to ask 'Why am I reading this?'. In other words, try to be explicit about your criteria for selection.

Evaluating the literature

When the use of published studies helps to inform actual practice, the term 'evidence-based medicine' is used. As in the analysis of an individual paper, the process of drawing conclusions must carefully reflect the limitations of the research being reviewed. The critical appraisal and reflection skills described in the first part of this book must now be used on several papers. But there are some new skills which involve finding common themes between articles as well as identifying discrepancies and discussing why they may have arisen. The process of identifying the main ideas related to a topic is a major theme in this second section of the book.

Illustrating the process of topic-based review

The process of evaluating the literature is illustrated in this book by a number of topics. By the time this book is published, it is inevitable that some of these 'hot' topics will have become luke warm or cold and that new evidence will have emerged. But that doesn't matter. The intention is to illustrate the process of using the literature rather than to write a series of review articles.

Systematic reviews

There is an emerging academic movement which has established guidelines for reviewing the literature (Chalmers and Altman, 1995). You may wonder why we did not use systematic reviewing as a starting point. The reason is that, although academically sound, the skills involved in systematic reviewing can be cumbersome and are sometimes frustrating for the beginner in the face of data presented in a non-systematic way. They are more appropriate for the researcher than for the practitioner who is 'reading for information'. Once you have made a start, however, you will probably find that critical reading becomes rapidly addictive and an important part of your continuing professional development. If so, you may want to refine your skills and the logical next stage is to tackle the systematic approach to reviews (Fullerton-Smith, 1995).

In the chapters which follow we will be concerned with the process of reviewing and evaluating the literature. As we are doing this based on 'reading for information' rather than for research, we do not spend time discussing our search strategies, but simply state what it was about the articles which made us choose them. Purists will not like this. However, search strategies make fairly dull reading. Our main intention is to illustrate how easy it can be to get useful information from a small number of articles and how reflection can relate this to practice.

A hot topic framework

It may not be necessary to use a formal systematic approach when making a start on reading about a topic, but some sort of framework is nevertheless helpful. In the next short chapter, we suggest an easy starting point which may help you when selecting what to read and how to organize the ideas in the literature.

Box 10.6 gives a summary of the stages in the critical reading of a topic.

Box 10.6 Summary of the stages in the critical reading of a topic.

1 Identify the topic, e.g. from a clinical problem.
2 Identify what you already know about the topic (including uncertainties) and identify what else you need to know.
3 Arrange a literature search.
4 Select what to read making criteria explicit.
5 Evaluating the literature, summarizing what you have read, drawing conclusions to inform practice, and making explicit any limitations or uncertainties.

REFERENCES

Baker, M., Maskrey, N., and Kirk, S. (1997) *Clinical Effectiveness and Primary Care*. Oxford: Radcliffe Medical Press.

Bradley, C. (1992) Uncomfortable prescribing decisions: a critical incident study. *British Medical Journal*, **304**, 294–296.

Bradley, C. (1996) Turning anecdotes into data – the critical incident technique. *Family Practice*, **9**, 98–103.

Chalmers, I., and Altman, D.G. (1995) *Systematic Reviews*. London: BMJ Publishing Group.

Fullerton-Smith, I. (1995) How members of the Cochrane Collaboration prepare and maintain systematic reviews of the effects of health care. *Evidence Based Medicine*, **1**, 7–8.

Greenhalgh, T. (1997) *How to Read a Paper: The Basics of Evidence Based Medicine*. London: BMJ Books.

Havelock, P., and Schofield, T. (1996) Learning consultation skills. In: *Professional Development in General Practice* (Pendleton, D. and Hasler, J. eds), pp. 36–50. Oxford: Oxford University Press.

Jones, R., and Kinmonth, A. (1995) *Critical Reading For Primary Care*. Oxford: Oxford University Press.

Minghella, E., and Benson, A. (1995) Developing reflective practice in mental health nursing through critical incident analysis. *Journal of Advanced Nursing*, **21**, 205–213.

O'Dowd, T. (1993) Critical incident analysis: cases and patterns. In: *Medical Audit in Primary Health Care* (Lawrence, M. and Schofield, T. eds), pp. 149–154. Oxford: Oxford University Press.

Pendleton, D., Schofield, T., Tate, P., and Havelock, P. (1984) *The Consultation: An Approach to Learning and Teaching*. Oxford: Oxford University Press.

Pietroni, R., and Millard, L. (1996) Portfolio based learning. In: *Professional Development in General Practice* (Pendleton, D. and Hasler, J. eds), pp. 81–93. Oxford: Oxford University Press.

Robinson, L., Stacy, R., Spencer, J., and Bhopal, R. (1995) Use of facilitated case discussion for significant event auditing. *British Medical Journal*, **311**, 315–318.

Sackett, D., and Haynes, R. (1995) On the need for evidence based medicine. *Evidence Based Medicine*, **1**, 5–6.

Sackett, D., Richardson, W., and Haynes, R. (1997) *Evidence-based Medicine; How to Practise and Teach EBM*. London: Churchill Livingstone.

Schon, D.A. (1983) *The Reflective Practitioner*. New York: Basic Books.

Silverman, J., Kurtz, S., and Draper, J. (1996) The Calgary–Cambridge approach to communication skills teaching 1: agenda-led outcome-based analysis of the consultation. *Education for General Practice*, **7**, 288–299.

11

Hot topic framework

When thinking about hot topics it helps to consider in what ways the published literature may be able to throw light on the subject in question. But even before diving into the literature in search of goodies, it is worth remembering that some of the most important ideas are already part of your working knowledge, even if you are not fully conscious of all of them (Schon, 1983). Therefore we include a number of elements in a hot topic framework which starts with 'Working knowledge' and has the mnemonic 'WILMA' (Box 11.1).

Box 11.1 Hot topic framework: WILMA.

1 **W**orking knowledge
2 **I**ndividual papers
3 **L**atest findings
4 **M**odels
5 **A**ction plan

We will discuss each of the components of the framework briefly in turn.

WORKING KNOWLEDGE

An essential starting point is to reflect on what you already know about a topic from your general experience at work. This can be surprisingly hard to do because it sometimes means making explicit ideas and knowledge which you take for granted. Further reading may make it easier to identify the assumptions upon which your clinical approach is based and may even disprove some of them. Nevertheless, we believe that a quick review of your own 'key ideas' is a useful starting point before 'hitting the literature'.

One reason for reflecting on your own practice is that it will help you to identify what you would like to find out from a literature review and help you to be appropriately selective in what you read. This reflective component is crucial if what you read is to be really useful. We will therefore use 'reflection stops' in each of the chapters which follow. Sometimes a specific question will follow from analysis of a critical incident or you may need information to inform a guideline or to help set standards for audit purposes. On other occasions, a more general enquiry may be driven simply by curiosity. It is still worth asking yourself what it was that sparked your curiosity because very often that will help in defining more precisely what you need to know.

INDIVIDUAL PAPERS

In many areas a single paper will be widely quoted and will be perceived as 'essential reading'. Why one paper rather than another achieves such status is a fascinating question which has generated endless speculation. Suffice it to say that it is usually fairly easy to spot the most quoted paper by a quick glance at the introduction and discussion sections of one or two review articles. Sometimes an exceptional review article can itself become the 'most quoted paper' by drawing together different aspects of a topic in a unique or particularly helpful way. It is definitely worthwhile finding the original article and trying to speculate on why it is so often quoted. Questions to ask are summarized in Box 11.2.

LATEST FINDINGS

Sometimes the 'latest findings' come from general practice research but very often quantitative evidence comes from trials carried out in hospitals. Such studies can generate important changes in our understanding of disease and this may be important for primary care. The extent to which findings may be generalized from one setting to another has been a major focus of Chapter 6. Consideration of the

---

Box 11.2 Why is paper 'x' so much quoted?

Questions to ask might include:

- Was there a new idea or concept?
- Did the study challenge received wisdom?
- Did the study provide final evidence of what had previously been a clinical hunch?
- Was there an immediate implication for primary care?
- Was there a resource or management implication?
- Do you find it as interesting as others have done? Why?

---

type of patient selected and whether similar effects might be expected outside the confines of a carefully controlled study should be part of the critical appraisal of such papers.

We find it helpful to give latest findings a separate category in the framework, because it highlights the need to search for the most recent evidence. Without this, it would be easy for guidelines to become 'set in stone'. There is a large lag period between the publication of important research findings and their implementation in practice (Haines and Jones, 1994). Awareness of the latest evidence is an important first step.

MODELS

We use the term 'models' very loosely; it can encompass many different aspects of how care is delivered and organized as well as ideas which help explain data of relevance to primary care. It is given a separate category in our framework because we believe it is always worthwhile reflecting on the ideas and assumptions behind practice and on how these change with time.

To be really useful, a model should be capable of generating hypotheses which can be tested.

Articles contributing ideas about models are sometimes based on qualitative research where investigators seek to describe the process of care without necessarily influencing it with an intervention. The description does not usually involve numbers and may include behaviours and what they mean to individuals. There is a strong and emerging methodology in this area which derives mainly from the social rather than the physical or biological sciences (Jones and Kinmonth, 1995). The approach is complementary to the quantitative one and there is an increasing recognition of its value (Mays and Pope, 1996). Research of this kind helps to provide an explanatory framework, new hypotheses or new light on a subject. This often has a more creative feel to it than the paper which sets out to test a hypothesis or provide important quantitative data. The point is, of course, that both types of approach are valuable and the types of information they provide are complementary.

Models of care may also be compared in a more traditional way: for example, a randomized controlled trial of the effects of self-monitoring of peak flow in asthmatics. Not all models are useful; if a model seems highly complex or counter-intuitive, it is worth asking why it has been developed and whether it is really needed.

We have included 'models' as a separate category as a reminder that not all research is quantitative and that even when it is, there are ideas behind the numbers.

Patients' perspectives

Models of health care may need to reflect the patient's perspective. Descriptions of this are often qualitative in nature. Studies may address many aspects including:

- Involvement of patients in the management of their own illness.
- Factors affecting compliance.
- Patients' views on quality of care issues.
- Patient groups.
- Communication between patients and health care staff.

ACTION PLAN

The final phase of critical reading is a return to reflection, so that conclusions can be drawn from the evidence and ideas in the literature. The extent to which they help with the problems which you identified in the initial stage of reflection ('Working knowledge') can be assessed. This might include asking some further questions:

- Have I asked the right question?
- Have new questions arisen following reading and reflection?
- Have I selected appropriate articles to read?
- What new or emerging evidence is there?

Then an action plan can be devised which might address some of the following elements:

- a need to ask further questions or read different articles;
- a need to audit an aspect of current practice or to set standards for practice;
- a need to make immediate changes in practice together with plans for evaluating change.

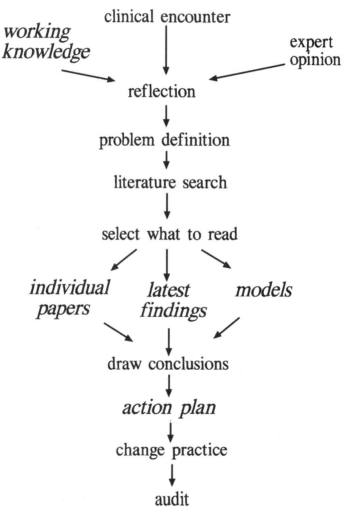

Figure 11.1 A literature review in the context of working knowledge, individual papers, latest findings, models and action plans.

USING WILMA

Figure 11.1 shows how the components 'working knowledge', 'individual papers', 'latest findings', 'models' and 'action plan' fit into a typical literature review generated after a clinical encounter.

We find the framework helpful because it makes one aware of the types of contribution specific publications can make. Simply asking 'What do I know, what problems can I identify and how could the literature help?' are powerful first questions in critical reading. In the chapters which follow, this framework will be used to illustrate the ways in which a few key papers can illuminate a topic and provide evidence to inform clinical practice.

REFERENCES

Haines, A., and Jones, R. (1994) Implementing the findings of research. *British Medical Journal*, **308**, 1488–1492.

Jones, R., and Kinmonth, A. (1995) *Critical Reading For Primary Care*. Oxford: Oxford University Press.

Mays, N., and Pope, C. (1996) *Qualitative Research in Health Care*. London: BMJ Books.

Schon, D.A. (1983) *The Reflective Practitioner*. New York: Basic Books.

12

Asthma in adults

WHY IS THIS A HOT TOPIC?

Despite the fact that much is known about the pathophysiology of asthma and its treatment, both morbidity and mortality remain high. The incidence of asthma appears to be rising and a significant number of patients still go undiagnosed (Frank *et al.*, 1996). Most GPs and practice nurses are commonly involved in managing asthmatics. Because the guidelines for management of asthma in children and adults differ in important respects (British Thoracic Society, 1993), we shall concentrate in this chapter on adults with asthma.

Since 1990, there has been a shift towards providing more asthma care in general practice and the model of a nurse run asthma clinic has been widely adopted.

The stimulus to review this as a hot topic might come from a critical incident, such as the death of a patient from acute asthma. Alternatively, a pharmaceutical adviser from the Health Authority may have visited and noted that your prescribing costs are rather high or low compared with regional and national averages. Or you might have done an audit of asthmatics and found only a few have a documented peak flow rate (PFR).

Reflection stop

Before reading on, pause for a few minutes and reflect on what are the main issues for asthma care within your own practice. Make a short list and then compare what you have written with the areas we have chosen to focus on: see 'Working knowledge' and 'Why the papers were chosen' below.

We will follow our basic framework for approaching a hot topic.

Box 12.1 Hot topic framework.

1 Working knowledge
2 Individual papers
3 Latest findings
4 Models
5 Action plan

WORKING KNOWLEDGE

Many practitioners are familiar with the presentation of both acute and chronic asthma. Before considering what the literature has to say about various aspects of this topic, it is worth doing a quick test of your own knowledge of the signs of acute asthma (Box 12.2).

Box 12.2 Task about acute severe asthma.

Task

British Thoracic Society Guidelines (1993, revised 1997) for the management of acute asthma in adults describe:

● Four signs of severe asthma;
● Six signs of life-threatening asthma.

What are they? Write a list before reading on. The answers are given in Box 12.3.

Box 12.3 Signs of acute severe asthma (from Guidelines for the management of asthma (British Thoracic Society, 1993)).

Four signs of severe asthma

- Unable to complete sentences in one breath
- Respiratory rate >25 per minute
- Heart rate >110 per minute
- PFR <50% predicted or best

Six life-threatening features

- PFR <33% predicted or best
- Silent chest
- Cyanosis
- Bradycardia
- Hypotension
- Exhaustion or confusion

Prophylaxis

Our working knowledge also recognizes the great value of prophylactic therapy and there are guidelines for chronic as well as acute asthma (British Thoracic Society, 1997). Some patients seem reluctant to use a 'preventer' and this may partly be a problem with the 'deferred gratification' involved: 'relievers' give quick relief when used correctly but 'preventers' do not give any sensation of efficacy at the time of use. There is a challenge to educate patients about the benefits of 'preventers' for those with moderate or poor control.

The other challenge is to find the most appropriate device for an individual patient and to check inhaler technique. The latter is often forgotten or omitted, particularly when there is time pressure in a clinic. This topic has recently been reviewed (Jackson and Lipworth, 1995) and will not be discussed in detail here. Many asthmatics do not use inhalers properly in public (Keeley, 1993), taking a quick and furtive puff, although perfect technique may be demonstrable in the clinic. The stigma attached to asthma, perhaps being perceived as a sign of weakness, may be part of the explanation for this.

In this chapter we are going to focus on some specific areas which we have identified as our own priorities and where the literature may illuminate our working knowledge:

- How to improve care.
- How to assess morbidity.
- Self-management plans.
- Prescribing as a measure of quality of care.
- Nurse-run clinics.

These may well not be the same areas as you have identified after personal reflection. Nevertheless, our hope is that the process of critical appraisal of papers relevant to these topics will illustrate an approach which you may wish to use in making an action plan for your own practice (see the end of this chapter).

WHY THE PAPERS WERE CHOSEN

A classic paper is our starting point (Keeley, 1993). This much quoted review article documents the main issues for asthma care in general practice. We will summarize the main recommendations made by Keeley.

One of the first points made by Keeley is that if you ask open questions like 'How is your asthma?', you will nearly always get the answer 'fine'. To get a more accurate assessment of how things are some specific closed questions are useful, like 'do you suffer from attacks of wheezing during the night?'. A morbidity index using three simple questions has been developed and this is the second paper discussed (Jones *et al.*, 1992).

The third paper looks at the next logical step: providing general practitioners with feedback about patients' self-assessments of symptom severity in an attempt to improve care (White *et al.*, 1995).

Next, we consider two papers on self-management plans (Charlton *et al.*, 1990; Grampian Asthma Study of Integrated Care, 1994a) because these seem to have become very popular. Are they just the latest fashion or is there really any good evidence that involving patients in managing their own disease alters the outcome? The debate about whether self-assessment should be by symptoms or by peak flow recordings is discussed. Figure 12.1 shows a typical peak flow meter.

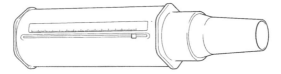

Figure 12.1 A peak flow meter.

Under the heading 'latest findings', we look at two papers from east London. The first looks at prescribing and quality of care (Naish, Sturdy and Toon, 1995). This article was chosen because the ratio of prophylactic to bronchodilator treatment is a simple index which is now being widely used. The second paper describes the effects of a practice-based educational intervention on the process of asthma care (Feder *et al.*, 1995). It was chosen partly because an improvement in prescribing was demonstrated and partly because it used a form of 'educational outreach' which seemed both appropriate for and acceptable to primary care teams.

Finally, we will come to 'models' and here we will look at two models of care which have been much discussed: nurse-run clinics (Jones and Mullee, 1995) and integrated care (Grampian Asthma Study of Integrated Care, 1994b).

INDIVIDUAL PAPERS

How to achieve better outcome in treatment of asthma in general practice (Keeley, 1993)

This paper has been much quoted as a highly influential review article. Before reading our summary of the article, try the task in the Reflection stop box.

> **Reflection stop**
>
> 'Reducing morbidity from asthma will depend on improvements in the provision of primary care for this condition.'
>
> Make notes on this statement before reading on.

Background

Poor organization of care and the false beliefs held by many practitioners are major obstacles. Here we will summarize Keeley's eight main points:

1 *Practitioners fail to identify symptoms.* An open-ended question 'How's your asthma?' usually elicits the reply 'Fine' whereas asking specific closed questions about how often patients have woken at night with cough or wheeze or how often work or school have been missed gives a much more useful measure of outcome.

2 *Practitioners think that regular use of bronchodilators is satisfactory treatment.* Many patients are on repeat prescriptions of these and using lots. British Thoracic Society guidelines suggest that if you need a reliever more than once per day, you should be on a preventer too. Many prescribe two reliever inhaler packs for each preventer, whereas good control might imply that you should need only one reliever for every two preventer units.

3 *Practitioners believe that inhaled steroids may be dangerous and are reluctant to prescribe effective doses.* There is no good evidence for growth retardation: effects of poorly controlled asthma on growth are more striking. Doubling the dose at the start of an attack or a bad cold will often stop it becoming severe and patients need to know when to do this and when to reduce the dose after an attack.

4 *Practitioners think that high doses of bronchodilators may be dangerous in an acute attack.* False. A single nebulizer dose is equivalent to about 25 metered dose puffs and this is often needed. 10–20 puffs every 4 hours via a large volume spacer is good treatment. If needed more often than 4 hours, medical help should be sought. Help should also be sought if PFR falls below 50% of best and if oral steroids are needed.

5 *Practitioners do not check whether patients can use their inhalers properly.* Poor technique is very common and 'almost no one uses their inhaler properly in public'. Check technique at each visit and encourage to use best technique at all times.

6 *Practitioners do not make enough use of large volume spacers.* These are cheap, deposit much more of a dose in the lung and retain their effectiveness in an acute attack. Figure 12.2 shows a typical spacer device.

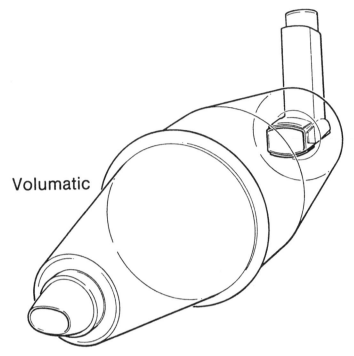

Figure 12.2 Large volume spacer.

Spacers also reduce prescribing costs by basing treatment on the much cheaper metered dose inhalers (MDI). Dry powder devices should 'only occasionally be needed' for daytime bronchodilation of patients who cannot use an MDI.

7 *Practitioners fail to ensure that patients are given consistent advice.* Different doctors and nurses give different messages which can be confusing. It is important to reach a consensus and to be consistent.

8 *Practitioners often make too much fuss about mild asthma.* Asthma varies a lot in its severity both between people and within an individual over time. We need to be more patient-centred, finding out about fears, e.g. asking specifically about worries over steroid side-effects. Often, health professionals respond to non-compliance by threatening patients with the consequences of bad asthma: this is rarely helpful and often alienates patients. Guidelines may lead to a lot of fuss about mild disease if not tailored to the level of an individual's disability.

Critical comment

Keeley hits the nail on the head with every point he makes and we have unashamedly summarized his main arguments. It is hard to criticize what he has written. In terms of spotting and articulating the problems, no one has done better. The only criticism might be in the title; there is an implication that outcome will be improved if these problems are corrected, but there is no indication about which of the eight should be of greatest priority or of what evidence for improved outcome might exist. A title such as 'How to improve the quality of asthma care' would have made no tacit assumptions about improved outcomes, which need to be demonstrated empirically.

We will return to the difficulty of showing improved outcome later when looking at the article which provides feedback to doctors of patients' self-assessment of symptom severity (White *et al.*, 1995).

Targeting asthma care in general practice using a morbidity index (Jones et al., 1992)

There is a high morbidity from asthma which has been shown in a number of community surveys (see Box 12.4).

Box 12.4 Typical findings from primary care surveys.

- Up to half of patients wake wheezy at least once per week.
- One-third have missed work or school in the previous year due to asthma.
- A quarter avoid physical activities because of asthma.

The authors of this paper developed an index on the basis of a questionnaire study. This had found three simple questions which could identify those with high morbidity and the index was significantly associated with lung function test results. The three questions are shown in Box 12.5.

Box 12.5 Questions for a morbidity index for asthma (Jones *et al.*, 1992).

1 Are you in a wheezy condition at least once per week?
2 Have you had time off in the last year because of asthma?
3 Do you suffer from attacks of wheezing during the night?

The morbidity questionnaire was sent to 853 asthmatics in a single group practice. The population was roughly split into thirds by this index. The term 'high morbidity' was used for those with two or more questions answered in the affirmative (moderate morbidity = only one affirmative; mild morbidity = none). Interestingly, 7% of those who had been labelled as asthmatic but believed they no longer had asthma were in the high morbidity group and 10% of those with asthma but on no current treatment were in the high morbidity category. Use of the index revealed that 2.5% of the practice list reported high morbidity and the authors pointed out that 'this is still too high a number for individual proactive care from doctors and nurses to be easily provided in the context of a busy general practice'. Nevertheless, use of this index may provide a way of aiming education and treatment at those most at need. For example, if self-monitoring of peak flow were to be targeted at a subgroup of more severe asthmatics, it might be helpful to use such a morbidity index.

Critical comment

The validity of the index could be judged in a number of ways. Reference is made to previous work where the index 'has been shown to correlate with lung function' but the strength of the correlation is not discussed. Perhaps the 'face validity' is enough justification for using it: it makes sense that the more questions answered in the affirmative, the worse the asthma is likely to be. The division into approximate thirds in this population also makes intuitive sense; if there is a continuous variation from good to poor control, categorization into 'high', 'medium' and 'low' morbidity seems reasonable. But it would be useful to know how often the classification got it right or wrong according to other criteria (such as peak flow) and whether similar results are obtained in other practices. In other words, the morbidity index is being proposed as a screening instrument and, as with all screening instruments, the more that is known about validity, reliability, sensitivity and specificity, the better.

Using information from asthma patients: a trial of information feedback in primary care (White et al., 1995)

This study used questionnaires, repeated at 6-monthly intervals over 2 years, to assess patients' self-reporting of symptoms, use of medications and attendance at the practice or hospital for asthma. Practices were randomly allocated to the control group, where this information was simply collected and an intervention group where the information was fed back to the primary care team in a number of ways, including inserts into individual patient records. The researchers felt that 'a key issue in the under-treatment and under-diagnosis of asthma may be ... lack of awareness of the morbidity experienced by their asthma patients'. They found that 45% of patients reported breathlessness at least once per week and less than half of these were using inhaled steroids, so there should have been plenty of room for improvement. Both groups improved over the course of the study but there were no differences in outcome between the intervention and control groups. The overall improvement may have been a Hawthorne effect, simply due to participating in a study about asthma which is likely to have a motivating effect on both doctors and patients. However, the feedback itself made little difference despite the fact that patient-derived information 'should be among the most powerful that could be used in the clinical setting' and seemed to be 'intrinsically powerful'. The authors noted that they had not attempted to alter the process of care by providing guidelines for the use of the information. There may also have been an issue of ownership: 'the motivation to collect and distribute the information came from the researchers. Individual practices did not request it, did not choose the information to be collected and did not decide on the way it should be presented or used'. This emphasizes that audit is not just about data collection; information alone will not be enough. To be successful in bringing about change, 'primary care teams first have to undergo the process of identifying their goals and then choosing the tools to help achieve them'.

Critical comment

This study presents an important 'negative' result. The authors started from a viewpoint which regarded patient-derived information as intrinsically powerful but realized by the end of the study that they had paid insufficient attention to the context and process of care. Interventions need to include guidelines for practitioners on how to use such data and the views and priorities of those providing care need to be addressed. The authors became aware of these problems and one of the strengths of their paper is in spelling out the need for strategic planning to develop processes within which information can be used. This clearly has broad implications for many aspects of care, not just in the field of asthma. The other strength is the further demonstration of the potential for improvement, with so many symptomatic patients on less than optimal therapy. There can be a bias in the selection of papers for publication, with positive findings more often reported than negative ones ('publication bias'). It is particularly good to see a paper published which has important implications despite a result which was negative in terms of the authors' initial hypothesis.

Self-management plans

The use of self-management plans has been heavily promoted in the last 5 years. Patients are educated so that they are able to take more responsibility for their own condition by initiating changes in their own treatment according to an individualized protocol which has been agreed in advance. An example of the type of plan which might be used is given in Box 12.6.

Evaluation of peak flow and symptoms only self-management plans for control of asthma in general practice

This study (Charlton *et al.*, 1990) compared two different types of plan: one was based on symptoms (e.g. 'if you get a cold, use your bronchodilator two puffs every four hours ... if you wake with wheezing at night, double the dose of inhaled steroids . . .') and the other was based on home peak flow measurements (similar to the one shown in Box 12.6). One hundred and fifteen patients attending a nurse-run asthma clinic were studied and the design was randomized (see Figure 12.3).

Box 12.6 Example of 'asthma treatment plan'.

Asthma treatment plan

NAME

YOUR BEST NORMAL PEAK FLOW RATE IS:

YOUR RELIEVER INHALER IS CALLED:

YOUR PREVENTER INHALER IS CALLED:

1 When you feel normal, continue usual treatment:
   - reliever when required plus preventer twice daily
   If you get a cold or your chest feels tight:
   - use your reliever up to two puffs every 4 hours as required
2 If your peak flow falls to less than 70% of normal (less than ....):
   - use your reliever – two puffs every 4 hours
   - double your dose of preventer for the number of days it takes to return to normal
   - continue on this increased dose for the same number of days
   - then return to normal treatment
3 If your peak flow falls to less than 50% of normal (less than ....):
   - start oral prednisolone (red prednisolone e/c 5 mg tablets: take 8 daily) and contact your GP
   - continue this dose for the number of days required to return to normal

All were on prophylactic therapy prior to the study. Both plans led to significant reductions in the number needing to see a doctor and in the number needing a course of oral steroids. Interestingly, there was no significant difference between the two groups and the authors concluded that teaching patients the importance of their symptoms and the appropriate action to take when their asthma deteriorates is the key to effective management of asthma. Simply prescribing peak flow meters without a system of self-management and regular review will be unlikely to improve patient care.

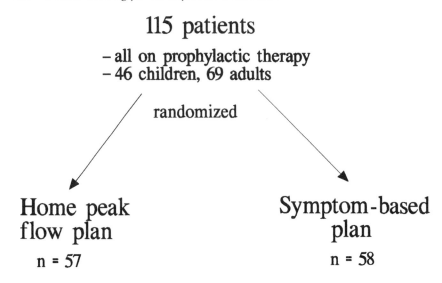

Conclusion: no significant difference in symptom control

Figure 12.3 Summary of study (Charlton et al., 1990).

Critical comment

The conclusions of this study have some similarities with the paper on feedback of symptoms to the primary health care team in that once again there was an improvement in both groups during the course of the study and there did not seem to be any clear benefit from an intervention. Here, the use of peak flow meters gave no better results even though one might have expected that the extra information they provide should be intrinsically useful. Note that:

- the sample size was small;
- the groups were not matched;
- there is the problem of a small but important subgroup who do not accurately perceive symptoms of impending severe asthma;
- type 2 error might have applied (failure to detect a real difference).

This study provoked a lot of debate. Hospital chest physicians, who tend to see a different case-mix with a higher proportion of more severe cases of asthma, argue strongly in favour of using PFRs as the objective basis of self-management plans. For some of these patients, changes in PFR may occur earlier than symptoms: different patients tolerate different degrees of bronchospasm, so symptoms may, in a few patients, be insufficiently sensitive as a guide to severity.

Effectiveness of routine self-monitoring of peak flow in patients with asthma

This paper (Grampian Asthma Study of Integrated Care, 1994a) was a report from the Grampian Asthma Study of Integrated Care (GRASSIC). This important project is reported in three separate papers: the other two are concerned with integrated versus conventional care and with enhanced versus conventional education.

Patients who did not already own a peak flow meter were randomized to self-monitoring of peak flow or to conventional monitoring. The results showed no difference in use of broncho-dilators, use of oral steroids, number of GP consultations or number of admissions after a year. There was no improvement in morbidity based on symptoms of asthma or measures of anxiety and depression in those given peak flow meters accompanied by guidelines for self-management. The authors concluded that routine prescribing of peak flow meters is unlikely to reduce morbidity or mortality.

The authors also reported on a subgroup: patients whose asthma was too severe for them to take part in integrated care between GP and hospital. They were maintained on conventional hospital care only. Those who had a peak flow meter showed a significant increase in the (appropriate) use of oral steroids. The overall conclusion was that self-monitoring of peak flow should probably be targeted at patients whose asthma is more severe or more unpredictable.

Critical comment

This study provides further evidence that routine prescribing of peak flow meters is unlikely to reduce overall morbidity or mortality. It also highlights the potential for differences in case-mix between patients seen in hospital and those seen in a general practice asthma clinic. Once again, this shows the importance of how 'cases' are selected and how careful one has to be in extrapolating results from one context to another.

It is important not to throw the baby out with the bath water; this result does not mean that peak flow recording is not important in the assessment of acute asthma, nor that a self-management plan based on peak flow may not be useful for those with severe or 'brittle' asthma. General practitioners with an interest in asthma already appear to use such plans for patients with severe symptoms which makes the design of randomized trials difficult (Hoskins *et al.*, 1996).

The two studies reviewed here concentrate on two related aspects of self-care: peak flow monitoring and self-management plans. Both of these patient-centred approaches seem appropriate for at least some patients with asthma, even though clear benefits have yet to be demonstrated in randomized controlled trials. It can be hard to perform such trials because many asthmatics are already self-monitoring to some degree and some doctors who volunteer for participation may be operating 'enthusiast bias' and this may confound results (Hoskins *et al.*, 1996).

LATEST FINDINGS

Appropriate prescribing in asthma and its related costs in East London

This paper (Naish, Sturdy and Toon, 1995) looked at the ratio of prophylactic to bronchodilator prescribing using prescription prescribing authority data for all general practices in a Health Authority area of East London. Practices approved for asthma surveillance and training practices were found to have higher ratios, indicating they were more likely to be following British Thoracic Society guidelines. These practices also had higher asthma drug costs. The cost data need to be interpreted with caution, since some are expressed as cost per prescribing unit which is related to list size and may therefore reflect inaccuracies such as 'ghosts'. One advantage of using the prophylactic bronchodilator ratio is that for this measure at least, the use of a ratio cancels out the list size denominator.

The authors commented that 'good clinical practice and cost consciousness do not necessarily go together. Pressure to reduce drug costs therefore may not increase the cost effectiveness of prescribing; indeed it may do the opposite'.

Critical comment

This study was unique in investigating all the practices within a single health authority area and making comparisons based on a simple index of quality of prescribing. The fact that training practices and practices approved for asthma surveillance have higher ratios provides support for the use of the ratio as a marker of quality of prescribing because these factors have 'face validity as likely to be markers for good prescribing'. The authors point out that the ratio is a relatively crude index of appropriateness of prescribing. However, that does not necessarily reduce its usefulness and it has the huge advantage of simplicity. The cost data also make sense because prophylactic inhalers are expensive, despite the caution in interpretation urged by the authors. The take-home message is that relatively simple analysis of prescribing data can give useful information to an individual practice which is interested in auditing this aspect of asthma care.

Do clinical guidelines introduced with practice-based education improve care of asthmatic and diabetic patients?

This randomized controlled trial in East London general practices (Feder *et al.*, 1995) is also discussed in the chapter on diabetes. The study used small group teaching methods to introduce guidelines. The 'educational intervention' consisted of three lunchtime meetings; introducing the guidelines and structured records for either diabetes or asthma, reviewing the clinical content of the guidelines and finally auditing some notes of patients 6 months later. Each practice received one set of guidelines, but provided data on management of both conditions after 1 year. Guidelines improved the recording of all seven variables on the diabetes prompt card. In the asthma practices, the difference between intervention and control practices was marginal, with only one of six variables (checking inhaler technique) being significantly better recorded. However, in both sets of practices there were big improvements in asthma recording during the study. It was postulated that the more complex nature of the diabetes review might have been a larger hurdle for a practice and might have had an indirect effect on asthma care. The main finding of significance to the asthma part of the study was a definite improvement in the quality of prescribing (a higher prophylactic bronchodilator ratio in the asthma practices compared with the diabetes practices). The authors point out that this is the first demonstration of changes in prescribing resulting from a guideline in British general practice.

Critical comments

If one accepts the validity of the prophylactic bronchodilator ratio as a crude measure of quality, this study has shown an improvement in prescribing following the introduction of guidelines.

A major strength is the randomized controlled design. The authors point out that valuable data might have been collected if there had been a further control group of practices receiving no guidelines at all and that this would have helped to assess the strength of the Hawthorne effect whereby involvement in the implementation of one set of guidelines might have had a beneficial influence on recording of variables in both conditions (i.e. the control condition as well as the intervention condition). However, such a control group would have increased the complexity and size of the study and important findings emerged even without it.

One of the most significant features of this study was the educational intervention itself. It is important that the practice based methods of dissemination were led by peers and were found to be acceptable to a wide range of practices. This may provide a useful model for implementation of guidelines in other areas. The components of 'educational outreach' used in this study are summarized in Box 12.7.

Box 12.7 Educational outreach (Feder *et al.*, 1995).

- Use small group methods.
- Focus on a specific group of clinicians.
- Define clear educational objectives.
- Establish credibility.
- Stimulate active participation.
- Use concise graphic educational material.
- Highlight and repeat key messages.
- Provide reinforcement by follow-up.

This approach contrasts with the study discussed above which provided feedback on patient morbidity without providing guidelines and without seeking the views of the primary care team in an interactive way (White *et al.*, 1995).

MODELS

In the last 10 years, the main model of primary asthma care to emerge has been proactive, nurse-run care in mini-clinics and we will consider a good review article on this topic (Jones and Mullee, 1995). At the same time, others have been considering whether shared care might be an effective option: the second paper discussed here will be from the Grampian Asthma Study of Integrated Care (GRASSIC) group (Grampian Asthma Study of Integrated Care, 1994b).

Proactive, nurse-run asthma care in general practice reduces morbidity: scientific fact or medical assumption? (Jones and Mullee, 1995)

The authors start by quoting evidence from the hospital setting which has shown that proactive care improves outcome for patients with asthma. They also refer to an important paper (Charlton *et al.*, 1991) which followed-up 112 patients attending a nurse-run clinic and found significant reductions in the numbers of acute courses of oral steroids, acute nebulizations and days lost from work. Unfortunately, because this was primarily an audit, there was no control group, so it is hard to say to what extent the nurse-run clinic was instrumental in the improvements which were noted. To address this difficulty, a prospective study was performed comparing two similar practices, with one practice developing a nurse-run clinic (the intervention practice) and the other continuing traditional reactive care (the control practice). Thus the design was a prospective, interventional, non-randomized, controlled trial. Despite considerable time and resources, the trial was unable to find significant differences in outcome between the two groups of patients. The authors found this disappointing and their discussion of the methodological problems with this sort of pragmatic research is illuminating. They highlight four main points:

1 The study was a comparison between two single practices and so numbers were relatively small. In addition, 30% of patients dropped out mainly through moving away. This may mean that a real difference was present but that the study was not powerful enough to detect it (a type 2 error, or false negative result).

2 The control practice was already operating good asthma care with a higher proportion of patients on prophylactic therapy throughout the study. This shows the difficulty in providing a good control group in a non-randomized design. It might have been easier to show a benefit in less well-advanced practices 'but gaining cooperation from such practices is often difficult'.

3 The patients studied had mild asthma, so there was limited scope for improving morbidity.

4 Confidential interviews revealed that the reception staff in the intervention practice felt ambivalent about the new asthma clinic and it is possible that this may have influenced the disappointing outcome. They also noted that it took 6 months for the new system to actually start and that considerable time, enthusiasm and resources were needed. This has implications for the successful management of change in general practice.

Critical comments

The discussion of the problems of proving the advantage of one model of care is very helpful. The authors' main conclusion was that the study had 'illustrated that benefits in lowered morbidity for patients in a practice are not immediate nor easy to achieve or demonstrate'. This is why many studies choose to look at secondary outcome measures, such as number of peak flow measurements recorded reflecting delivery of care, rather than primary outcome measures such as morbidity.

What is most interesting is the observation that the group of patients selected had only mild asthma. Perhaps practices and researchers should be focusing more on patients with poorly controlled asthma. If such patients were studied the potential for improvement might be higher. One of the problems is that some are reluctant to attend, may have difficulty in coping with the health care system or may deny the existence of asthma (Charlton *et al.*, 1991). The stigma of asthma may be of particular importance here (Sibbald, 1989).

Integrated care for asthma: a clinical, social and economic evaluation
(Grampian Asthma Study of Integrated Care, 1994b)

The work of the GRASSIC study on peak flow measurement has already been discussed. This paper reports the results of their comparison between conventional and integrated care. The patients recruited were already attending a hospital outpatient clinic regularly and so probably had moderate or severe asthma. About 10% of patients were considered too severe for randomization by their chest physician. The remainder were randomized into two groups. The intervention group were seen annually in the hospital and had interim reviews every 3 months by their GP who collected a questionnaire which had been sent in advance to the patient. This was forwarded to the consultant together with the details about consultations, medication and peak flow. An updated computerized record was returned to the GP with advice from the consultant about any changes in the management plan. The control group continued with 3-monthly outpatient attendance.

In some previous studies of shared care in diabetes poorer outcomes were reported, but in this study no significant differences were found in a variety of measures, ranging from symptoms and peak flow to psychological dysfunction. The authors conclude that shared care is clinically effective and a realistic option for patients with moderately severe asthma. Although, three quarters of patients wished to continue with integrated care, the authors noted a 'credibility gap' in the control group where patients were less likely to want to take the opportunity of shared care. These were individuals who had become long-term attenders at outpatient clinics: 'the general perception of hospital consultants as experts and general practitioners as "generalists" is neither easily nor quickly dispelled'.

Critical comments

It is interesting to note that in this study, the lack of a difference was regarded as a major success whereas in several studies already mentioned, a non-significant difference was regarded as a failure. The reason is clear from the authors' discussion in which they highlight the evidence from the field of diabetes where poor supervision and worse control resulted after discharge of patients into the community setting. Thus, they were pleased to show a lack of deterioration in shared care patients as a positive result! It seems likely that the care taken to ensure effective communication between patient, GP and consultant with computer-generated, user-friendly forms was a key component.

This is an important result because it focuses on patients with relatively severe asthma and shows that integrated care is both clinically effective and popular with patients. GPs also found the scheme acceptable (Van Damme *et al.*, 1994). The amount of enthusiasm and work needed to set up and run such a system should not be underestimated. Although the authors do not present details of their 'economic evaluation', they claim a small saving both for the hospital and for the GP and a greater saving for patients.

CONCLUSIONS

A number of common themes emerge from the articles considered. Some relate specifically to research methodology and some specifically to asthma. An example of a methodology issue is the fact that improvements were noted in the control group in three separate studies and these improvements made it hard to find a significant difference due to the intervention. This was a feature of the paper on feedback to doctors of patient-derived information (White *et al.*, 1995), of the paper on guideline implementation for asthma and diabetes (Feder *et al.*, 1995) and also in the paper on nurse-run care versus conventional care in two different practices (Jones and Mullee, 1995). This emphasizes firstly the importance of having a control group in the study design. Secondly, it raises the question of why control groups so often show an improvement. At least part of the reason may be the fact that they are part of a study which is in itself highly motivating (the Hawthorne effect).

What have we learned from reviewing these articles which might inform our working knowledge of asthma? The main points are summarized in Box 12.8.

The final point is particularly important – both clinicians and researchers should probably concentrate more of their energy on those with moderate and severe asthma, reflecting one of the key messages of Keeley: don't make too much fuss about mild asthma.

Perhaps the single most important conclusion is that the classification of asthma severity is a useful starting point in deciding

Box 12.8 Main conclusions.

- Asthma is common and morbidity is high
- Severity can be assessed by asking a few simple closed questions as well as by using peak flow measurement
- The benefits of self-management plans are hard to show in those with mild or moderate asthma
- Many patients like self-management plans as they promote autonomy
- The benefits of a nurse-run clinic are hard to demonstrate but there are no reasons to believe they are any less effective than conventional care
- Integrated care is a feasible option for many patients with moderate asthma
- A significant proportion of asthmatics under-use health services. This may in part reflect the stigma attached to the condition
- Preventers are under-used and this is an example of the 'implementation gap' which may be closed by an educational intervention with subsequent audit
- Educational outreach, based on small group methods with active participation of targeted clinicians, is an acceptable and effective method of implementing guidelines
- Don't make too much fuss about mild asthma

whether a patient is suitable for prophylaxis, home peak flow recording, intensive education in a nurse-run clinic or hospital referral. Both history, current symptoms and peak flow recording will help. Once such classification becomes incorporated into practice, it may be easier to achieve and demonstrate improvements in outcomes.

ACTION PLAN

At the beginning of this chapter, you were asked to identify the main issues of relevance to asthma care in your own practice. Reflect again on these; they may be very different from the example we have chosen to discuss in this chapter.

Reflection stop

- Which of your questions remain unanswered?
- Which further sources of information do you feel you need?
- What type of audit of asthma care might be most helpful?
- What changes have you thought of?
- What resources are available?
- Who else should be involved?

After reflection, try discussing your ideas with colleagues, a mentor or an audit facilitator. The implementation of evidence-based medicine can sometimes be hard (Haines and Jones, 1994). It is worth thinking about general issues of managing change as well as how any obstacles to change may be overcome (Spiegal *et al.*, 1992).

REFERENCES

British Thoracic Society (1997) The British Guidelines on asthma management. *Thorax*, **52**, Supplement 1, 1–21.

Charlton, I., Charlton, G., Broomfield, J., and Mullee, M. (1990) Evaluation of peak flow and symptoms only self-management plans for control of asthma in general practice. *British Medical Journal*, **301**, 1355–1359.

Charlton, I., Charlton, G., Broomfield, J., and Mullee, M. (1991) Audit of the effect of a nurse run asthma clinic on workload and patient morbidity in a general practice. *British Journal of General Practice*, **41**, 227–231.

Feder, G., Griffiths, C., Highton, C., Eldridge, S., Spence, M., and Southgate, L. (1995) Do clinical guidelines introduced with practice-based education improve care of asthmatic and diabetic patients? A randomised controlled trial in general practice in East London. *British Medical Journal*, **311**, 1473–1478.

Frank, P., Ferry, S., Moorhead, T., and Hannaford, P. (1996) Use of a postal questionnaire to estimate the likely under-diagnosis of asthma-like illness in adults. *British Journal of General Practice*, **46**, 295–297.

Grampian Asthma Study of Integrated Care (1994a) Effectiveness of self-monitoring of peak flow in patients with asthma. *British Medical Journal*, **308**, 564–567.

Grampian Asthma Study of Integrated Care (1994b) Integrated care for asthma: a clinical, social and economic evaluation. *British Medical Journal*, **308**, 559–564.

Haines, A., and Jones, R. (1994) Implementing the findings of research. *British Medical Journal*, **308**, 1488–1492.

Hoskins, G., Neville, R., Smith, B., and Clark, R. (1996) Do self-management plans reduce morbidity in patients with asthma? *British Journal of General Practice*, **46**, 169–171.

Jackson, C., and Lipworth, B. (1995) Optimizing inhaled drug delivery in patients with asthma. *British Journal of General Practice*, **45**, 683–687.

Jones, K., and Mullee, M. (1995) Proactive, nurse-run asthma care in general practice reduces morbidity: scientific fact or medical assumption? *British Journal of General Practice* **45**, 497–499.

Jones, K., Charlton, I., Middleton, M., Preece, W., and Hill, A. (1992) Targeting asthma care in general practice using a morbidity index. *British Medical Journal*, **304**, 1353–1356.

Keeley, D. (1993) How to achieve better outcome in treatment of asthma in general practice. *British Medical Journal*, **307**, 1261–1263.

Naish, J., Sturdy, P., and Toon, P. (1995) Appropriate prescribing in asthma and its related costs in East London. *British Medical Journal*, **310**, 97–100.

Sibbald, B. (1989) Patient self care in acute asthma. *Thorax*, **44**, 97–101.

Spiegal, N., Murphy, E., Kinmonth, A., Ross, F., Bain, J., and Coates, R. (1992) Managing change in general practice: a step by step guide. *British Medical Journal*, **304**, 231–234.

Van Damme, R., Drummond, N., Beattie, J., and Douglas, G. (1994) Integrated care for patients with asthma: views of general practitioners. *British Journal of General Practice*, **44**, 9–13.

White, P., Atherton, A., Hewett, G., and Howells, K. (1995) Using information from asthma patients: a trial of information feedback in primary care. *British Medical Journal*, **311**, 1065–1069.

13

Diabetes

WHY IS THIS A HOT TOPIC?

Since the 1990 contract, specific payment has been made for providing care for diabetics in general practice. Shifting care from hospital to the community has gained increasing support since the description of 'mini-clinics' (Thorn and Russell, 1973) and patients appear to like the primary care setting (Murphy, Kinmonth and Marteau, 1992). There is a challenge to provide high quality care in a local setting. In addition, district-wide registers of diabetics are being set up and multidisciplinary approaches are being encouraged. The St Vincent Declaration (1989) provides an internationally agreed set of aims for diabetes care.

The stimulus to review this as a hot topic might come from a critical incident such as a patient going blind in one eye due to proliferative retinopathy which has been missed or from a proposal from a local consultant that a shared care scheme might be a good idea. Alternatively, an audit may have highlighted an aspect of care which is often missed within the practice, for example checking the feet or the eyes.

Reflection stop

Before reading on, pause for a few minutes and reflect on what are the main issues for diabetes care within your own practice. Try to formulate the areas you are interested in and questions to which you would like an answer. Compare your list with the areas we have chosen to focus on in this chapter: see 'Working knowledge' which includes 'Why the papers were chosen' below.

Box 13.1 Hot topic framework.

1 Working knowledge
2 Individual papers
3 Latest findings
4 Models
5 Action plan

WORKING KNOWLEDGE

Practitioners vary in their interest in this chronic disease and in the knowledge and skills they possess. Some confine themselves to managing type 2, non-insulin dependent patients while others accept all diabetics. Some prefer not to take responsibility for eye checks and involve other professionals in these. Some prefer to 'share care' with a hospital clinic. Others fear they may become de-skilled because one of their partners has taken on the care of all the diabetics in the practice. Some practitioners are truly working in a mini-clinic with the support of an on-site dietician, a chiropodist and specialist nurses. Others are isolated and struggling without a multi-disciplinary team to provide such support, often with the brunt of the work being borne by one person, usually the practice nurse. Diabetes can affect every part of the body and because of the numerous complications, attention to detail is an essential component of care.

Accompanying such variation in practice are questions about the quality of care provided, the continuing education of those involved, the provision of adequate resources and the outcomes for patients with this disease.

WHY THE TOPICS WERE CHOSEN

In this chapter we will choose five areas, each of which is illustrated with critical reference to one or two important articles. Along with each area, we have included the main question which prompted us to start reading.

1 Screening for diabetes: is it worthwhile?
2 Eye checks: can GPs perform them effectively?
3 Glycaemic control and microvascular complications: what is the link?
4 Shared care: how could it work?
5 The patient's perspective: what do they think about general practice-based care?

Before considering these it is worth noting an area which has *not* been chosen for discussion because of limitations of space. This is the use of interventions to reduce cardiovascular risk in type 2 diabetics which is important because up to 75% will die from vascular causes. Attention to smoking, blood pressure, lipids and the use of aspirin for secondary prevention are all as important as assessing glycaemic control (Mather *et al.*, 1996). Evidence for the effectiveness of such interventions are generally extrapolated from findings in non-diabetic patients, but since risk factors operate similarly, and since the absolute risk is so much higher in diabetic patients, this is probably justified (Mather, 1996).

WHY THE PAPERS WERE CHOSEN

It is important to consider screening for diabetes because diabetes is a common condition and because testing urine samples is a relatively simple procedure. But how does this screening test stand up to closer scrutiny? Mant and Fowler's paper was chosen because it clearly explains the limitations (Mant and Fowler, 1990).

The aspect of diabetes care which GPs feel most uneasy about is checking the eyes. Retinopathy is both common and treatable and several papers have documented the poor performance of GPs in fundoscopy. The study from Bath was chosen because it is brief and widely quoted (Finlay *et al.*, 1991).

The link between poor glycaemic control and microvascular complications has been recognized for some time. A large and recent study in the USA has provided evidence that intensive therapy to improve glycaemic control does reduce the incidence of such complications (The Diabetes Control and Complications Trial Research Group, 1993). The implications of the DCCT trial for type 1 diabetics will be discussed.

Several models of care will be briefly mentioned. There has been a useful review article, an Occasional Paper from the RCGP, about shared care which will be considered in more detail (Greenhalgh, 1994a).

Finally we will look at the patient's perspective, evaluating a piece of qualitative research (Murphy, Kinmonth and Marteau, 1992).

INDIVIDUAL PAPERS

Screening for diabetes

Urine analysis for glucose and protein: are the requirements of the new contract sensible?

About 2% of the population have diabetes but only 1% know it. There are a large number of undiagnosed patients with type 2 diabetes in the community. An important paper by Mant and Fowler (1990) points out some of the problems with unselective routine urine testing, such as the cost and the poor quality control in some clinical settings. The yield from screening depends partly on age. Consider the figures in Table 13.1 which are fictitious, but typical of the sorts of results obtained. Calculate the positive predictive value of the test for each age range before reading on.

The positive predictive value is the proportion of those who have a positive result on the screening test (i.e. glycosuria present) who

Table 13.1 Age stratified figures for the prevalence of diabetes

Age	Number tested	Number (%) positive for glycosuria	Number (%) with previously undiagnosed diabetes
<40	1000	20 (2)	2 (0.2)
40–59	1000	40 (4)	10 (1)
>60	1000	60 (6)	20 (2)

truly turn out to have the condition being sought (diabetes on a glucose tolerance test). The predictive value is only 10% (2 out of 20) in those under 40 but rises to 25% (10 out of 40) of those aged 40–59 years and 33% (20 out of 60) of those over 60 years. Thus significant numbers of undiagnosed diabetics may be picked up by primary care screening programmes, particularly where the elderly are targeted.

Critical comment

The value of this cannot be judged for certain until there is evidence to show that early detection improves outcome, although there are already good reasons to believe this to be the case. It is very important to be aware that a large number of false positives will be generated particularly in the young and middle-aged groups and practitioners will have to work hard to minimize the anxiety generated by this.

Can general practitioners screen their own patients for diabetic retinopathy?

Fundoscopy skills of general practitioners are variable. This recent report (Finlay *et al.*, 1991) suggested very poor sensitivity (proportion of affected individuals correctly identified) when compared with a hospital consultant and this applied not only to the whole group of patients but also to those with 'sight-threatening retinopathy' (Box 13.2).

Critical comment

The first point is that this study looked at GPs who had been given no special training. Although this may apply to many, it does not apply to all. It also raises the question about how easily training can improve clinical performance and there is some evidence that benefits can be achieved (Stead, Dudbridge and Hall, 1991). Nevertheless, the results of the Bath study indicate the need for further work in this area and for quality assurance schemes.

There is the second issue of what should be the gold standard for the clinical diagnosis of retinopathy. Should this be a consultant

---

Box 13.2 Poor results of untrained GP fundoscopy.

Bath study (Finlay *et al.*, 1991)
21 GPs studied; only one practice had a diabetic mini-clinic.
GPs performed dilated fundoscopy on 300 eyes.
Checked by consultant ophthalmologist using direct ophthalmoscopy (reference standard).

Specificity
Measured on individuals without the condition.
Proportion correctly identified as 'normal'.
Bath study: specificity of GPs 86%.

Sensitivity
Measured on those with the condition.
Proportion correctly identified as being affected.
Bath study: sensitivity of GPs 55%.
Applied to 'all retinopathy' as well as 'sight-threatening retinopathy'.

Bath study conclusions
● Screening by own GP not effective.
● Mini-clinics might produce better results.
● Feedback from consultant over cases where opinions differed would provide educational opportunity.

---

using a slit-lamp? This was not the case in this study. The main question for practitioners is whether to check the eyes themselves or refer to the diabetic clinic or the eye clinic. It is difficult to answer without data comparing groups of hospital doctors from the diabetic and eye clinics as well as trained GPs. It may be that consultants in the diabetic clinic are very good at detecting retinopathy, but without the data this assumption cannot be proved.

Some practices use their local optician for retinopathy checks but there have been few formal assessments of optician's skills. Alternative approaches include the use of a retinal camera with photographs checked by a consultant, but these have generally produced disappointing results (Leese *et al.*, 1993).

The Wessex survey

A survey in Wessex identified some even more basic problems with the delivery of eye care (Alexander and Canning, 1995). See Box 13.3 for a summary.

Box 13.3 Summary of the Wessex survey.

- 50% of GPs in Wessex responded to questionnaire.
- 60% were checking acuities.
- But few were aware of technique of pinhole correction.
- 76% performing fundoscopy.
- But half were not dilating the pupil.

LATEST FINDINGS

DCCT trial

Read the following abstract and then spend 10 minutes making notes on the following question: 'Consider the implications for diabetes care in the UK'.

Title: The effect of intensive treatment of diabetes on the development and progression of long-term complications in insulin-dependent diabetes mellitus (DCCT, 1993).

Abstract

Background: Long-term microvascular and neurologic complications cause major morbidity and mortality in patients with insulin-dependent diabetes mellitus (IDDM). We examined whether intensive treatment with the goal of maintaining blood glucose concentrations close to the normal range could decrease the frequency and severity of these complications.

Methods: A total of 1441 patients with IDDM – 726 with no retinopathy at base line (the primary prevention cohort) and 715 with mild retinopathy (the secondary intervention cohort) – were randomly assigned to intensive therapy administered either with an external insulin pump or by three or more daily insulin injections and guided by frequent blood glucose monitoring or to conventional therapy with one or two daily insulin injections. The patients were followed for a mean of 6.5 years, and the appearance and progression of retinopathy and other complications were assessed regularly.

Results: In the primary prevention cohort, intensive therapy reduced the adjusted mean risk for the development of retinopathy by 76% (95% confidence interval, 62 to 85%), as compared with conventional therapy. In the secondary intervention cohort intensive therapy slowed the progression of retinopathy by 54% (95% confidence interval, 39 to 66%) and reduced the development of proliferative or severe nonproliferative retinopathy by 47% (95% confidence interval, 14 to 67%). In the two cohorts combined, intensive therapy reduced the occurrence of microalbuminuria (urinary albumin excretion of >40 mg per 24 hours) by 39% (95% confidence interval, 21 to 52%), that of albuminuria (urinary albumin excretion >300 mg per 24 hours) by 54% (95% confidence interval, 19 to 74%), and that of clinical neuropathy by 60% (95% confidence interval, 38 to 74%). The chief adverse event associated with intensive therapy was a two-to-threefold increase in severe hypoglycaemia.

Conclusions: Intensive therapy effectively delays the onset and slows the progression of diabetic retinopathy, nephropathy and neuropathy in patients with IDDM.

Critical comments

We will consider implications in note form and divide our comments into 'generalizations' and 'consequences'.

Generalizations

Subjects

- Clearly defined group.
- But possible that USA patients may be different in important ways, e.g. health consciousness or compliance with therapy.
- It would be very dangerous to extend the results to type 2 diabetics who make up the main case-load in UK primary care.

Similar questions about such patients are being asked in separate studies, for example the United Kingdom Prospective Diabetes Study (UKPDS Group, 1995).

Setting

- This was a randomized trial of intensive care.
- The Hawthorne effect might apply: being in a study may have increased the efficacy of the intervention.
- This was a hospital-based study; it might give different results in patients recruited in the community.
- It would be difficult to arrange such care universally. Could the NHS cope?

Results

- Reduced complications: retinopathy, nephropathy, and neuropathy.
- Large effect was shown.
- Main side-effect: hypoglycaemia. The trial would present the most optimistic picture though no figures are given in the abstract. This must be of serious concern as hypoglycaemia can be fatal.

Consequences

Costs

Time, pumps, monitoring, workload, training.

Patients

Acceptability, compliance, autonomy: 'Good control or a happy life' (Alberti, 1992).

It is likely that this evidence will lead both doctors and patients to be more obsessional about glycaemic control, but the awaited evidence of the continuing UK study of type 2 patients will have more importance for the majority of patients seen by their GP. There is potentially a conflict with patient freedom in pressing for stricter regimes; involvement of the patient in making an informed choice will be crucial.

MODELS

About 25% of diabetics receive no organized care. The quality of the care provided, both in hospital clinics and in general practice is seldom carefully evaluated. Dr Pat Thorn, the physician in Wolverhampton who pioneered Mini Clinics in the 1970s (Thorn and Russell, 1973), is often quoted as having said 'If I had diabetes, I wouldn't attend my own clinic'.

The key to successful diabetic care is organization. This applies equally to the hospital and general practice settings. The first step is to have a comprehensive register of diabetics and the second is to have an efficient recall system. Protocols for care include the use of flow charts to encourage the attention to detail required for monitoring a complex chronic disease. With such arrangements, an interested GP may look after his own diabetic patients in ordinary surgery time. This is described as 'organized personal care' (Foulkes *et al.*, 1989).

The idea of a general practice mini-clinic was pioneered in the 1970s and has become increasingly popular. One possible disadvantage of such systems is that often one partner takes on the responsibility for diabetes care and this may involve some 'deskilling' of other partners within a practice. There is also a risk that a more disease-centred approach may lead to a decline in holistic care. In other words, the nurse may see to the blood pressure, the chiropodist to the feet and the doctor to the eyes. It may be easier to forget about the 'whole person' with such a model of care. On the other hand, advantages may include a consistent and organized team approach with the provision of care at a single visit. This is also consistent with effective use of a practice's time and resources.

Hospital versus general practice care

A study from the West Midlands (Parnell, Zalin and Clarke, 1993) looked at the clinics of 11 general practices and compared case notes with two hospital clinics. There was no evidence that general practice clinics were overall less successful than hospital clinics at monitoring for complications. The study noted variations in the quality of care between the different practices and between the two hospitals. The importance of audit as a way of improving care was emphasized for both hospital and GP settings.

Critical comments

This was a retrospective audit of case notes and hence dependent on the accuracy of the medical records. Possible differences in the populations attending hospital and GP also make interpretation of such studies difficult, particularly if the outcome of care is to be assessed. Showing the frequency with which the eyes or feet are checked is one thing, but assessing the quality of the examination is another and assessing the impact on health is even more difficult.

A prospective controlled study in a deprived area of East London found a big improvement in the recording of key variables following a series of three educational lunchtime meetings in which locally developed guidelines were discussed in a small group setting (Feder *et al.*, 1995). In addition the use of a structured booklet to act as a prompt further improved recording. The effectiveness of these interventions was impressive. The authors point out that previously it had been widely believed that 'ownership' of protocols could only be achieved by being involved in writing them. Their work provides evidence of the powerful educational effect of carefully planned small group meetings.

The potential of general practice clinics to match or exceed the quality of care provided in hospitals has been shown in several studies, but this may depend on the care of selected patients in selected practices (Wood, 1990). The degree of support of such clinics varies enormously. This raises issues such as access to biochemical testing, dietician and chiropody services, and ophthalmology. It also places a heavy responsibility on practice nurses, many of whom have not had adequate education in this area. There is an English National Board course specifically designed for nurses undertaking diabetes care.

The Community Diabetes Specialist Nurse may be able to help a practice nurse set up and run a diabetic clinic as well as forming an important link between doctors and patients.

Another important issue is the potential for discontinuity of care in the hospital setting where junior doctors change jobs frequently.

Shared care

In a few centres, shared-care systems have been developed along similar lines to those used in obstetrics. This topic has been extremely well reviewed (Greenhalgh, 1994b). Shared care has been defined as 'the joint participation of hospital consultants and general practitioners in the planned delivery of care for patients with a chronic condition, informed by an enhanced information exchange over and above routine discharge and referral notices'. Greenhalgh summarizes the experience of several different groups who have developed shared-care schemes. Although 'each health district is unique in its demography, resources, health needs and local political climate . . ., some fundamental principles for successful shared care undoubtedly remain'. (See Box. 13.4.)

Box 13.4: Requirements for successful shared care (after Greenhalgh, 1994).

- Enthusiastic and committed personnel, e.g. community specialist nurse acting as facilitator.
- Teamwork with an egalitarian, multidisciplinary approach. Some early reports of shared care were really of 'dumped' care where a hospital consultant unilaterally discharged patients from a hospital clinic to unstructured GP care.
- Computerized register to prompt care and evaluate outcome, preferably across a whole district.
- Written guidelines of clinical care and its organization.
- A diabetes resource centre with responsibility for education of both patients and health professionals and aiming to empower both patients and primary care professionals.
- Clear channels of communication: exciting possibilities exist for making better use of existing channels (shared-care cards, regular letters) plus newer possibilities like electronic smart cards with computer-assisted care.

Some patients dislike seeing 'a different doctor every time' in hospital clinics and may dislike shared care for similar reasons. Patient motivation to use a shared-care card for 9 months of pregnancy is great but may not be so high for 20 or 30 years of a chronic disease. In addition successful shared care requires an enormous input in terms of planning and communication. An enthusiastic and effective multidisciplinary team is probably the key element for success in shared care.

Critical comments

The systematic review of shared care (Greenhalgh, 1994b) found no evidence from five randomized controlled trials of any benefit from shared care in terms of clinical outcome. An editorial in the *British Medical Journal* discusses the complexities involved (Sowden, Sheldon and Alberti, 1995):

1 It is hard to do randomized controlled trials as the definition of shared care varies from simply handing out a protocol to the GP through to more involvement in decision-making and information exchange.
2 In the field of asthma, the Grampian study of integrated care used a $2 \times 2 \times 2$ design to allow comparison of three components: level of education, use of peak flow self-monitoring and integrated versus conventional care. This shows the potential for finding out which aspects of care are most important for outcome and this type of design might usefully be applied to diabetes.
3 It is important to take into account consumer preference as quality of life and psychological wellbeing are important outcomes. These are not always consistent with good glycaemic control as tight control is associated with stricter regimes and more hypoglycaemic episodes. Such outcomes are important in evaluating shared care.

The importance of this last point goes beyond the confines of a clinical trial. Practitioners need to share responsibility for management with patients and must recognize that good glycaemic control is not the only important outcome. It could also be argued that if you do not have easy access to a skilled dietician (preferably on-site) and facilities for teaching self-monitoring, it is hard for either the practitioner or the patient to make a truly informed choice. Access to a dietician and the presence of an interested doctor have both been shown to be associated with better glycaemic control (Pringle *et al.*, 1993), so there is no room for complacency.

Evaluation of care

Most primary care initiatives are not properly evaluated. Two key components of the audit cycle tend to be missed. Firstly, the aims of a clinic must be made explicit and secondly, ideal standards must be set so that outcome measures for success can be selected. This may sound a daunting task but in one study, transfer of data to computer took very little time for practices undertaking structured care using a flow sheet (Tunbridge *et al.*, 1993). This can enable audit of both process of care (e.g. proportion with eye check or recent measurement of glycated Hb) and intermediate outcome of care (e.g. proportion with retinopathy or high glycated Hb). Such continuing audit is essential for improving quality of care and will hopefully, over time, lead to improvement in final outcomes such as amputation rate, prevalence of blindness and renal failure and death. These events being less frequent are difficult to interpret in the context of a single practice.

Patients' perspective

Patients like the easier access of general practice care and find the setting more acceptable than the 'cattle market' quality of some hospital clinics. The British Diabetic Association has produced a Patients' Charter which spells out the minimum standard of care which a diabetic should expect. This organization encourages patients' active involvement in their own condition. A recent study from Southampton (Murphy, Kinmonth and Marteau, 1992) compared patients' views of the service they received before and after the introduction of a diabetic mini-clinic. Patients were in favour of the proposals to start the clinic in general practice and this enthusiasm was sustained a year after the clinic was started. They saw the GP as being easier to talk to and better at listening than doctors in hospital diabetic clinics. They also perceived no significant difference in expertise compared with the hospital specialist.

Critical comment

Patients' perceptions can sometimes be flattering; the evidence suggests GP's skills at detecting retinopathy are limited although no direct comparison with hospital clinic staff has been made. However, it is clear that many patients do like the primary care setting and this piece of qualitative research uses quotes from patients to remind us why. It is worth noting that a working group of the World Health Organization and St Vincent Declaration Action Programme has been looking at ways of encouraging psychological well-being in people with diabetes and their families. One of their reports details ways in which satisfaction with treatment may be assessed using a validated eight-item psychometric questionnaire (Bradley and Gamsu, 1994). This sort of approach can give a quantitative assessment of satisfaction with treatment and may prove useful for those wishing to assess the effects of change in the provision of care.

Main concepts reviewed

The literature has provided evidence in a few key areas. Screening for diabetes and detection of diabetic retinopathy have been identified as particular problems. It is clear that many patients like the setting of general practice; if effective diabetic care is to be provided, audit must be part of the process, a multidisciplinary team approach is ideal and the organization of care must be carefully planned. Shared care offers the potential for a mix of the generalist and specialist approach, but needs equally careful planning and evaluation.

ACTION PLAN

The final phase of critical reading is a return to reflection, so that conclusions can be drawn from the evidence and ideas in the literature. The extent to which they help with the problems which you identified in the initial stage of reflection about diabetes ('Working knowledge') now need to be assessed. It may well be that your own questions have not been addressed or that the literature considered here may not have provided useful answers. If this is so, it is important to acknowledge it. In any case, it is worth asking some further questions (see Reflection stop box).

Reflection stop

- Which of your questions remain unanswered?
- Which further sources of information do you feel you need?
- What type of audit might be most helpful?
- What changes have you thought of?
- What resources are available?
- Who else should be involved?

An action plan can be devised which might address some of the following elements:

- a need to ask further or different questions;
- a need to read different articles;
- a need to audit an aspect of current practice;
- a need to make immediate changes in practice together with plans for evaluating change.

Start to formulate your own action plan now. Do not be put off if there still seem to be a lot of unanswered questions. Reflect on what are your priorities. An action plan does not have to be perfect or comprehensive: a 'good enough' plan is much better than no plan and if it is 'short and simple' it is more likely to be be lead to successful change.

REFERENCES

Alberti, K. (1992) Good control or a happy life? In: *Current Themes in Diabetes Care* (Lewin, I. and Seymour, C., eds), pp. 67–71. London: Royal College of Physicians.

Alexander, M., and Canning, C. (1995) A telephone study of diabetic retinopathy and the diabetes miniclinic in general practice: a regional study in Wessex. *Practical Diabetes*, **12**, 28–30.

Bradley, C., and Gamsu, D. (1994) Guidelines for encouraging psychological well being. *Diabetic Medicine*, **11**, 510–516.

Feder, G., Griffiths, C., Highton, C., Eldridge, S., Spence, M., and Southgate, L. (1995) Do clinical guidelines introduced with practice based education improve care of asthmatic and diabetic patients? A randomised controlled trial in general practice in East London. *British Medical Journal*, **311**, 1473–1478.

Finlay, R., Griffiths, J., Jackson, G., and Law, D. (1991) Can general practitioners screen their own patients for diabetic retinopathy? *Health Trends*, **23**, 104–105.

Foulkes, A., Kinmonth, A., Frost, S., and MacDonald, D. (1989) Organised personal care – an effective choice for managing diabetes in general practice. *Journal of the Royal College of General Practitioners*, **39**, 444–447.

Greenhalgh, P. (1994) Shared care for diabetes: a sytematic review. *Occasional Paper 67*, pp. 1–35. London: Royal College of General Practitioners.

Leese, G., Ahmed, S., Newton, R., Jung, R., Ellingford, A., Baines, P., Roxburgh, S., and Coleiro, J. (1993) Use of mobile screening unit for diabetic retinopathy in rural and urban areas. *British Medical Journal*, **306**, 187–189.

Mant, D., and Fowler, G. (1990) Urine analysis for glucose and protein: are the requirements of the new contract sensible? *British Medical Journal*, **300**, 1053–1055.

Mather, H., Cassar, J., Bloom, S., and Wise, P. (1996) *Diabetes Care in the Community: A Practical Guide*, 2nd edn. Wilmslow, Cheshire: Zeneca Pharmaceuticals.

Murphy, E., Kinmonth, A., and Marteau, T. (1992) General practice based diabetes surveillance: the views of patients. *British Journal of General Practice*, **42**, 279–283.

Parnell, S., Zalin, A., and Clarke, C. (1993) Care of diabetic patients in hospital clinics and general practice clinics: a study in Dudley. *British Journal of General Practice*, **43**, 65–69.

Pringle, M., Stewart-Evans, C., Coupland, C., Williams, I., Allison, S., and Sterland, J. (1993) Influences on control in diabetes mellitus; patient, practice or delivery of care? *British Medical Journal*, **306**, 630–634.

Sowden, A., Sheldon, T., and Alberti, G. (1995) Shared care in diabetes. *British Medical Journal*, **310**, 142–143.

Stead, J., Dudbridge, S., and Hall, M. (1991) The Exeter diabetic project: an acceptable district-wide education programme for general practitioners. *Diabetic Medicine*, **8**, 866–869.

The Diabetes Control and Complications Trial Research Group (1993) The effect of intensive treatment of diabetes on the development of long-term complications in insulin-dependent diabetes mellitus. *New England Journal of Medicine*, **329**, 977–986.

Thorn, P., and Russell, R. (1973) Diabetic clinics today and tomorrow: mini-clinics in general practice. *British Medical Journal*, **2**, 534–536.

Tunbridge, F., Millar, J., Schofield, P., Spencer, J., Young, G., and Home, P. (1993) Diabetes care in general practice: an approach to audit of process and outcome. *British Journal of General Practice*, **43**, 291–295.

UKPDS Group (1995) Relative efficacy of randomly allocated diet, sulphonylurea, insulin, or metformin in patients with newly diagnosed non-insulin dependent diabetes followed for three years. *British Medical Journal*, **310**, 83–88.

Wood, J. (1990) A review of diabetes care initiatives in primary care settings. *Health Trends*, **22**, 39–42.

14

Heartsink patients

WHY IS THIS A HOT TOPIC?

The feelings induced in practitioners by their patients form a major theme in British general practice following the work of Balint. Many different terms have been used to describe patients perceived as difficult, but 'heartsink' seems to be the most widely used, summarizing as it does the strength of feelings in a way which is lacking in descriptions such as 'problem patients'.

Communication is central to primary care and it has been found that difficulties arise in about 25% of consultations (Pendleton and Bochner, 1980). Only a small number of such difficulties will make the practitioner's heart sink, but when it does sink, the feelings induced can be strong and can influence communication with other patients, with colleagues and with family and friends. For these reasons, it is likely that heartsink patients will always be a hot topic as practitioners struggle to find effective ways of providing care while at the same time trying to understand and deal with their own negative emotions.

Michael Balint, the psychoanalyst who pioneered small group seminars to analyse general practice consultations during the 1950s and 1960s, pointed out that 'Because every therapy is based on an interplay between patient and doctor, it cannot really be understood if one restricts one's observations to the one or the other: the therapy happens not in the patient nor in the doctor but between the two of them' (Balint, 1964).

Although the term heartsink patient implies implicitly that the source of the problem is the patient, and is pejorative because of this, it is essential to remember that problems arise from an interaction between practitioner and patient and that the contribution of both to the relationship must be acknowledged.

Reflection stop

Pause for a moment and consider one or two patients you have seen recently who have made your heart sink.

● What was it about them which was difficult?
● Can you think of other patients where similar difficulties have arisen?
● What feelings did you experience?
● How have you dealt with such feelings in the past?
● Can you identify anything about your approach, attitude or life experience which may have made these consultations difficult?
● Finally, how do you think reading the literature might help in dealing with patients like these?

Make some brief notes before reading on.

We will be using the 'hot topic framework' and start with 'Working knowledge'.

Box 14.1 Hot topic framework.

1 Working knowledge
2 Individual papers
3 Latest findings
4 Models
5 Action plan

WORKING KNOWLEDGE

There are a number of ideas which can be derived from our working experience of heartsink patients and six main points are relevant here.

1 Heartsink patients are being defined by the effects they have on the practitioner and these can include feelings of:

- frustration, irritation, exasperation, anger, dislike, hatred;
- sadness, hopelessness, inadequacy;
- unprofessionalism because of the strong negative emotions felt.

Ellis (referring to 'dysphoria' induced by patients) describes the feelings as: 'feelings felt in the pit of your stomach when their names are seen on the morning's appointment list' (Ellis, 1986). The range of emotions is wide as indicated above and may include particularly a sense of humiliating failure and disappointment in oneself for having such 'unprofessional' feelings.

2 Many different types of behaviour can induce such feelings; if it was only one type, you might expect that we would all have gone on a simple course to learn the appropriate coping skills.

3 There are a few patients who manage to antagonize every practitioner they see, but there are probably an equal number who just 'get under the skin' of one particular practitioner and with whom other carers have no major problems. This raises the question of whose problem it really is.

4 Some patients go through a difficult phase, often related to life events, when they appear to make enormous emotional demands on those providing care. When circumstances change, they may no longer make your heart sink.

5 Heartsink patients may be hard to define but (like the elephant) you're pretty sure you know one when you see one. A heartsink patient is not the same as a frequent attender because many of the latter do not cause such strong antipathy. However, they do seem to consult frequently. They are also different from somatizers although some may have a tendency to somatization. Similarly, the term dysfunctional consultation may apply to some interactions with heartsink patients but may equally apply on particular occasions to patients with whom one has a relationship which is not characterized by a sense of heartsink. It may be best to regard these other terms as overlapping concepts which commonly form part of a heartsink doctor–patient relationship but which do not necessarily define it. Some, but not all, patients 'with a list' can cause a feeling of heartsink (Middleton, 1994). (Fig. 14.1.)

6 The concept of 'housekeeping' is appealing: health professionals can find it helpful to reflect on the feelings induced in them by

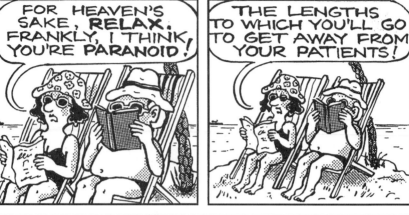

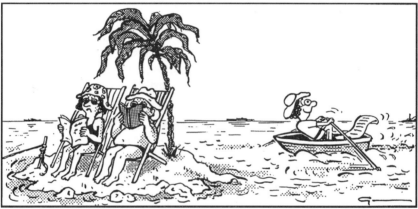

Figure 14.1 A patient with a list.

patients and should be able to deal with such feelings appropriately, without damage to themselves or others (Neighbour, 1987).

HOW CAN THE LITERATURE HELP?

Do you think that reading the literature can help in any way? Your gut reaction may be 'No' because the literature seems to be so 'academic' whereas this whole area is about dealing with strong emotions and also about communication. At the least, the literature may help by reassuring you that you are not alone in experiencing strong negative emotions. But it has the potential to do more than that; the experience and reflections of others can suggest very practical ways of coping and of developing skills which will enhance your professional practice.

Our working knowledge of heartsink patients can be illuminated by a number of different approaches, some using traditional methods to describe the epidemiology of heartsink patients and others developing ideas and models based on more qualitative observations. The tensions between these two types of approach were obvious to those working with Balint in the 1960s and remain in many ways unresolved. Here the intention is to use the best of both to throw light onto what we already know from working in general practice.

WHY WERE THE PAPERS CHOSEN?

Now let us consider what the literature has to say about heartsink patients.

1 Four stereotypes of 'hateful patients' were described by an American psychiatrist (Groves, 1978). This paper is widely quoted and provides a simple classification of some of the main sorts of behaviour which reliably upset clinicians. It also emphasizes the validity of the practitioner's feelings as diagnostic data: it is helpful to examine these feelings for managing the patient as well as for managing yourself.

2 A classic paper by O'Dowd describes the 'epidemiology' of heartsink patients in a single British group practice and is also widely quoted (O'Dowd, 1988). It shows how a team approach with some simple interventions can help.

3 A recent paper (Mathers, Jones and Hannay, 1995) focuses on the variation between doctors in numbers of patients reported as being heartsink, showing that it takes two to sink a heart and emphasizing, for a change, the practitioner's contribution in broad 'epidemiological' terms.

4 As a 'latest finding', we summarize a helpful article which provides a 'heartsink survival pack' (Mathers and Gask, 1995). The pack consists of strategies for somatizing patients, general approaches to problem consultations, coping skills and suggestions for group work.

5 Finally, under the heading models, we consider two books. The first introduces the concept of housekeeping (Neighbour, 1987). The second provides a model of straightforward and complicated

transactions (Norton and Smith, 1994). A distinction is made between the public domain, which includes the social roles adopted by practitioners and patients, and the personal domain where all the psychodynamic attributes that make up an individual are considered.

INDIVIDUAL PAPERS

Taking care of the hateful patient (Groves, 1978)

Groves points out that negative reactions to patients 'constitute important clinical data about the patient's psychology' and that emotional reactions 'cannot simply be wished away, nor is it good medicine to pretend they do not exist'. Rather such feelings can be used in an attempt to understand the patient and can facilitate appropriate psychological management. He confines his attention to patients who cause more than mild irritation: those 'whom most physicians would dread to treat' and defines four stereotypes of 'hateful patient' (Box 14.2). All have in common a great dependency on carers; an 'insatiable dependency'.

Box 14.2 Summary of Groves' classification.

1 Dependent clingers – will not take responsibility.
2 Entitled demanders – dissatisfied with service, excessive demands: 'I know my rights'.
3 Manipulative help rejectors ('nothing has worked').
4 Self-destructive deniers (e.g. deny risk factors).

Dependent clingers

Clingers make repeated requests for reassurance, explanation, tablets and all sorts of care. They are 'overt in their neediness' and see the physician as 'inexhaustible'. Early on such patients may express genuine gratitude, but to an extreme degree and the practitioner may feel powerful and special because of this. There may be flattery by the patient or even unconscious seduction. Later, when the demands for care are incessantly repeated, the practitioner may become exhausted. Groves uses the analogy of a mother's relationship with an unplanned, unwanted and unlovable child and points out that any attempt to refer the patient to a psychiatrist are usually interpreted correctly as rejection and doomed to failure. The best management is to inform the patient that the practitioner 'has not only human limits to knowledge and skill but also limitations to time and stamina'. In addition, it may help to take the initiative in arranging follow-up. The practitioner 'who begins to feel an aversion towards the patient should think of setting limits on dependency'.

Entitled demanders

These patients may feel equally needy but they express their need in an overtly hostile way, using intimidation, threats of litigation, devaluation and guilt induction. This is perceived by the practitioner as either pathetic or repulsive and often induces a wish to counter-attack. It may be hard for the practitioner to realize that such behaviour may be a way of preserving the self 'in a world that seems hostile or during an illness that seems terrifying'. Attacking the patient by denying their entitlement may be harmful; it is better to acknowledge the entitlement but redirect it towards the goal of good care. Groves points out that it is easy to get into fruitless debate with such patients and suggests the best approach is to assure the patient repeatedly that you will do your best to ensure that they get the best possible medical care.

Manipulative help-rejectors

'Unlike clingers, they are not seductive and grateful; unlike demanders they are not overtly hostile.' Instead, they return repeatedly saying that the treatment or plan suggested has not worked. They seem quite satisfied by this, sometimes smug. The more efforts the practitioner makes, the more pessimistic are the patient's reports. If one symptom improves, another 'mysteriously appears in its place'. What is really sought by the patient, probably unconsciously, is 'an undivorcible marriage with an inexhaustible caregiver'. The practitioner starts out anxious that a treatable condition may have been overlooked, then becomes irritated by the repeated appearance of a pessimistic patient. Finally, the practitioner may begin to doubt him- or herself and become depressed. Groves suggests that the correct intervention is to 'share the pessimism – to say that the treatment may not be entirely curative'.

Regular follow-up may be planned as a way of ensuring that the patient may begin to realize that if he loses his symptoms he will not necessarily lose his practitioner.

Self-destructive deniers

These are patients such as the alcoholic with oesophageal varices who continues drinking. They are profoundly dependent but 'have given up hope of ever having needs met. Such patients seem to glory in their own self-destruction. They appear to find their main pleasure in furiously defeating the physician's attempts to preserve their lives'. Groves points out that what one can do to help them is quite limited and that doctors usually respond with a wish that the patient will die 'and get it over with'. It may help the carers to recognize that the denier may actually wish to die. The wish to abandon the patient should be resisted and compassion found 'just as one does with any other patient with a terminal illness'.

Critical comments

It is important to remember that Groves was describing patients seen mainly in hospital practice and referred for psychiatric assessment which may have exerted selection bias on the sample to which he was exposed. In addition, his descriptions are of stereotypes; this is a powerful way of expressing what appear to be consistently linked attributes or types of behaviour, but may be misleading because reality is more complex than the stereotypes derived from it. There are no data which might enable us to know how often patients perceived as having dependency problems also have a tendency to reject help, for example. Groves recognizes this problem when he says 'At times, a single patient may epitomize more than one of these classes'.

Nevertheless, there may be value in a qualitative description such as this if the face validity is high; in other words if the description is found, at face value, to be true. Certainly, most in primary care can recognize the dependent clinger and the help-rejector as stereotypes which 'ring a bell'. We find it more difficult to think of really heartsink patients in the other two categories, entitled demanders and self-destructive deniers. However, recent work suggests that a specific category of heartsink patient may exist with a previously low consultation rate and a tendency to personality problems and episodes of self-harm in response to acute life events (McDonald and O'Dowd, 1991). It may be that these have something in common with the 'self-destructive denier' and their relative infrequency may make them harder to recognize.

The other way in which Groves' paper helps is in the advice he gives to practitioners to re-frame their roles. Lowering an aim of delivering 'perfect care' or stating the limits to consultation duration and availability can be liberating.

Finally, there is a major problem with the use of the term 'manipulative'. Linehan has pointed out the pejorative nature of this term (Linehan, 1993). She describes the great temptation to make an error of logic: to infer a behavioural intent from the effects of the behaviour. In other words, just because the professional feels manipulated does not mean that the patient intended to influence others artfully, shrewdly or fraudulently. 'Otherwise we would have to say that people in pain or crises are "manipulating" us if we respond to their communications of distress.' It would therefore be better if the simpler term 'help-rejector' were used to describe such patients in a less judgemental way.

Five years of heartsink patients in general practice (O'Dowd, 1988)

This paper reports an audit of the heartsink patients in a single practice and found that the number was smaller than anticipated from the strength of feelings induced: only 0.3% of the list size were in the heartsink category.

These patients were found to attend frequently (16 consultations per year compared with the average consultation rate of three), but they were not synonymous with the frequent attender as 20% had a lower consultation rate than another family member. There was a tendency to see many partners with a perceived potential for manipulation. The rate of missed appointments was high and the female : male ratio was 3:1.

One of a practitioner's greatest fears may be that his or her emotional response will lead to a missed diagnosis, that they will ignore the symptoms of a difficult patient 'crying wolf'. Although 30% of heartsink patients were found to have a serious medical diagnosis, fortunately there were few 'missed diagnoses'.

Over 5 years the number of heartsink labels fell by 30%. Studying the problem may have been part of the solution. The factors which seemed to help are summarized in Box 14.3.

Box 14.3 Factors which seemed to help (O'Dowd, 1988).

1 Obtaining more information about the patient and family.
2 Formulating a management plan even if clinically based.
3 Appointing a key worker.
4 Providing support for key practitioner from partners and staff.
5 Forming a contract, setting limits or confronting.
6 Admitting existence of negative feelings.

Outcomes were assessed after 5 years. Many patients had moved away, hence for some the outcome was uncertain. Some patients expressed their dissatisfaction and found another practice. Some seemed to have lost their 'problem' status. It was recognized that a few patients remained unlikeable and difficult to help.

Critical comments

This study was a small but unusual audit. It was unusual because it looked at a non-clinical subject. As an audit, it did not matter that doing the study was probably altering the behaviour of doctors and patients (the Hawthorne effect); in fact the interest provoked by the study may well have been a major factor in altering the practitioners' perceptions of when a patient was a 'heartsink', contributing to the fall in the number of heartsink labels used over 5 years.

Because the numbers were small and because of expected 'turnover' in the list, it is difficult to draw firm conclusions from the 5-year follow-up data. Even so, there were a few cases where the consultation rate declined and a 'truce' was thought to have been reached between doctor and patient. This raises the possibility that for some being a heartsink patient may be a temporary stage in a person's life experience and this idea has other evidence to support it (McDonald and O'Dowd, 1991). Whether changes in the patient's life or changes in the management strategy were more important cannot be judged from this study.

The paper describes how lunchtime meetings were arranged to discuss problem patients in a small group multidisciplinary setting and how 'the meetings stopped after six months because of pressure of time and doubt that the effort was worthwhile'. This is an important point because one of the crucial ingredients to success is teamwork and peer support which was, in this practice for this purpose at least, poorly sustained. The author pointed out that this inadvertently created two comparison groups; one group had been discussed in the meetings and the other group did not have specific management plans. Comparison between the groups must be limited because they were not formed by random allocation; indeed the 'worst' patients were discussed first in the planning meetings.

Nevertheless, the author noted a decline in the consultation rate of both groups which suggests that changes in the doctor's approach to heartsink patients in general may have been influential whether or not an individualized management plan had been made. The focus of the lunchtime meetings was in forming a management plan, but it is equally possible that the covert process of sharing and support was the truly important intervention. This was an audit and not designed to distinguish these two possibilities. Either way, it emphasizes the need for protected time and sustained enthusiasm to provide a multidisciplinary approach with proactive care.

Heartsink patients: a study of their general practitioners (Mathers, Jones and Hannay, 1995)

One practitioner's list of problem patients may not be the same as another's. This paper presented the results of structured interviews with 137 GPs in Sheffield; the number of heartsink patients reported in each interview was compared with the doctor's scores for general health, job satisfaction and self-reported experience of training in communication skills. The authors found that no doctor said they had not experienced heartsink patients. The number of patients reported varied from 1 to 50. The individual characteristics of doctors were associated with the number of heartsink patients they reported. Sixty percent of the variance could be accounted for by four variables which are shown in Box 14.4.

The authors concluded that 'the greater a doctor's perceived workload and job dissatisfaction, the more heartsink patients he or she is likely to report'. They went on to suggest that lessening or reorganizing workload may be a way to reduce the number of heartsink patients experienced. They also commented that: 'training in counselling skills might enable general practitioners . . . to reduce the number of heartsink patients they experience and their levels of perceived stress'.

Box 14.4 Doctor factors associated with perceiving higher numbers of heartsink patients (Mathers, Jones and Hannay, 1995).

1 Greater perceived workload.
2 Lower job satisfaction.
3 Lack of training in counselling or communication skills.
4 Lack of postgraduate qualifications.

Critical comments

This study is important in focusing on the practitioner's contribution to the experience of heartsink. The authors were able to gather important data which were analysed to see how much of the variance between doctors could be accounted for by measurable factors. It is important to note that 'explaining variance' does not imply causation. For example, complaining in an interview about a large number of heartsink patients and complaining about high workload might both be the result of a doctor with a low threshold for complaining. It does not necessarily mean that there is something about complaining which causes, directly or indirectly, the experience of heartsink. Similarly, it may be simplistic to assume, as the authors seem to be doing, that because higher perceived workload accounted for some of the variance, reducing workload will of itself reduce the proportion of patients perceived as 'heartsink'.

The link with communication and counselling skills is interesting and probably does have real implications because there is other evidence to suggest that such training may be effective (Bowman, Goldberg and Millar, 1992).

The main implication of this study, then, is to focus attention on the contribution of the practitioner to the 'troubling patient encounter' and this is related both to the need for skills training and also to the wider issue of 'burnout'.

LATEST FINDINGS

Surviving the 'heartsink' experience (Mathers and Gask, 1995)

The feeling of heartsink is often experienced as 'angry helplessness' and practitioners often feel they do not know what to do when such patients consult. This often boils down to lack of control, called 'helplessness in the helpers' by Adler (1972). The solution may be in part to recognize that practitioners' 'hearts often sink because they cannot control their patients, yet many patients . . . have a desperate need to be in control of something and the doctor patient consultation may be an easy target for those feelings'. Rather than enabling the practitioner to feel more in control, the authors wish to promote a 'more balanced, open and realistic view of what has happened in the consultation'.

A small one-day workshop was designed to give participants a greater understanding of the heartsink experience and to facilitate the development of coping skills. They describe a 'heartsink survival pack' with four components (Box 14.5).

Box 14.5 The heartsink survival pack (Mathers and Gask, 1995).

1 Skills for difficult consultations with a somatizing patient.
2 General strategies for difficult consultations.
3 Coping strategies.
4 Goal reassessment: a problem-solving approach for group discussion.

Skills for difficult consultations with a somatizing patient

The first stage is to make the patient feel understood by taking a full history including exploration of health beliefs, emotional issues and social and family factors. The second stage is to 'broaden the agenda' by giving honest feedback of the results of examination and tests, acknowledging the reality of the symptoms (crucial) and reframing the symptoms. This involves linking physical, psychological and life events in a tentative way leaving the patient room to negotiate. Thirdly, 'making the link' by giving the patient a simple explanation of how psychological distress can cause physical symptoms and test to see if the explanation is accepted.

General strategies for difficult consultations

These include:

a Clarifying current problems by summarizing them to the patient
b Making a problem list with the patient as a way of taking control of how time is spent and negotiating which problems can appropriately be tackled.
c Ventilation of painful or difficult feelings.
d Goal setting.
e Mutually agreed 'homework', as a way of testing the patient's capacity to change.
f Providing supportive feedback.

Coping strategies

a Share the difficulties with colleagues.
b Developing boundaries; making it clear to yourself and the patient what your professional role is and trying to work within that role. Sometimes practitioners are drawn beyond their usual boundaries in an attempt to help a particular patient; if such efforts are not valued by the patient, the practitioner can quickly become disillusioned and less effective than if clear professional boundaries had been maintained from the start.
c Challenging own attitudes. For example, some may have difficulty saying 'I cannot help you'. Letting go of a patient may challenge the way we see ourselves as providing care to all comers.
d Confronting hopelessness. It is often helpful to get an outside view as things may not be as hopeless as they feel.
e Accepting powerlessness; if there is little that can be achieved, one may have to accept one's own powerlessness: an example of where attitudes need to be challenged because healers often feel the need to be in control.

Goal reassessment: questions to ask in case discussion

a What is the problem? What am I hoping to achieve?
b What sources of support do I have access to?
c How realistic are my expectations of myself?
d How realistic are my expectations of my patient?
e Am I guilty of undervaluing what I have achieved so far?
f What is my plan of action now?

Critical comments

This article describes the benefits of a short workshop and gives excellent guidance on how to use a small group setting as a 'survival pack'. We have unashamedly summarized the main headings of this paper because it emphasizes the benefits of patient-centredness, including the value of eliciting health beliefs, acknowledging the reality and validity of symptoms even when a psychosomatic explanation seems likely and using techniques such as summarizing and writing problem lists as ways of promoting shared responsibility. In our view this is essential reading for all primary care practitioners.

What the article does not do is to provide a detailed analysis of the problems which a practitioner can bring to the consultation; it alludes to these in discussing how one might have to challenge and redefine 'how one views one's role'. The authors add 'a key coping strategy involves identifying and challenging these schemata and the "rules" may be largely unconscious until challenged in group discussion about a particular patient'. More could have been said about why practitioners often wish to be in control and what their needs are in a professional relationship. This is only a minor criticism because the aim of the paper was to provide a summary of practical skills for use by small groups; the authors may have assumed that detailed analysis of an individual practitioner's assumptions would be more appropriately explored in that setting than in the paper itself.

MODELS

There are many models of the consultation, but the one which is most helpful in the context of a heartsink patient is that of Neighbour (1987) because it includes a separate category 'Housekeeping', which highlights the doctor's feelings.

In *The Inner Consultation*, Roger Neighbour describes a handful of key processes within a consultation (Neighbour, 1987). These are called the 'five checkpoints' of the consultation (Box 14.6).

Housekeeping

The thumb of Neighbour's hand model is 'housekeeping' (Figure 14.2).

Box 14.6 Five checkpoints in the consultation (Neighbour, 1987).

1 **Connecting:** getting on the same wavelength as the patient.
2 **Summarizing:** a counselling skill which shows you have listened and clarified what the patient has said and have understood the reason for consulting you.
3 **Handing over:** giving the patient responsibility in the management plan and making sure he is happy with the outcome of the consultation.
4 **Safety netting:** planning with the patient for the unexpected helps to deal with uncertainty.
5 **Housekeeping:** being aware of your own emotions, how they have influenced this consultation and how they may influence subsequent ones. Looking after yourself. A consultation is not really complete until a practitioner has at least started this self-check process.

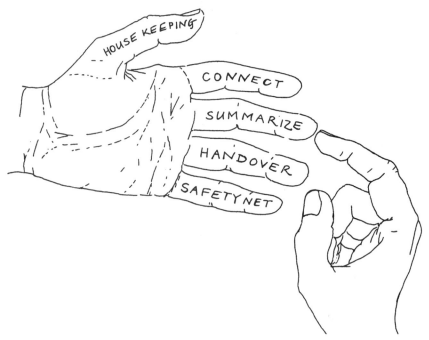

Figure 14.2 Five checkpoints of the consultation.

Apart from keeping yourself healthy, housekeeping can give very valuable insights into the feelings generated by a patient in other people and this may prove useful in understanding the problems presented and in helping the patient to deal with them.

Denial of emotional reactions

Neighbour points out the major issue of denial: we 'don't mind patients and psychoanalysts having unconscious needs, but not us, thank you very much'. Hence many practitioners deny their feelings or the relevance of those feelings and are certainly very reluctant to discuss them with others. However, the practitioner 'who is aware of all these needs and forces at work in him finds that knowledge of his own human frailty brings with it a deepening humility and compassion. He begins to feel safe without barriers . . . By knowing what passions govern him, yet remaining unafraid of them, they are subdued'.

Neighbour likens such self-awareness to housekeeping: minute to minute tidying is needed as well as regular spring cleaning. In other words one needs to be aware of one's feelings at moments within and between consultations as well as making longer term plans for things like regular holidays, rejuvenating hobbies, physical fitness and participating in professional support groups such as young practitioner groups or Balint seminars.

During the consultation

Neighbour divides the stresses of a consultation into two categories: 'extrinsic' and 'intrinsic'. Extrinsic stresses may be factors such as interruptions and sleep deprivation which are not directly related to the particular clinical interaction, but which can nevertheless have a damaging effect on it. Intrinsic stresses are those which 'arise as a result of your reactions, often irrational, to the particular patient who has inadvertently rubbed you up the wrong way'. These are the most interesting as they probably mediate the heartsink experience.

Telling the patient how you are feeling is not recommended unless you have had training and supervision in psychotherapy techniques and are planning to use the revelation of your feelings as a prelude to a therapeutic discussion. But Neighbour describes four other techniques and his description of them is summarized below.

1 **Spot the projection**

Sometimes patients remind us by chance of someone we dislike and we project our negative feelings onto the 'innocent' patient in a form of mistaken identity. The way to deal with it is firstly to recognize that it has happened and then to try to note a few specific features of the person in front of you which are dissimilar to the memory which has been evoked.

2 **Spot the stereotype**

Stereotypes reflect prejudices about certain categories or groups and can turn one's attention away from the specific qualities of an individual. Again, the first stage is to recognize that it is happening and the next stage is to look for some feature which does not fit in with the stereotype.

3 **'Here and now awareness'**

Techniques such as focusing your attention on your breathing can be helpful in crowding out unpleasant thoughts and associations. 'If you plant your feet on the ground, your head comes out of the clouds.' 'Do not try to alter your natural breathing or turn it into what you imagine relaxed breathing to be. Just notice the way it is.' Neighbour describes such techniques as 'quick centring' in restoring equilibrium.

4 **Adjust your muscle tone**

The basis of many relaxation techniques is to monitor and alter muscle tension, e.g. in the jaw, neck, shoulders and fists. 'Tense and then let go' techniques can be very effective.

Critical comments

Neighbour's 'inner consultation' model is unique in providing a major category, housekeeping, which specifically draws attention to the practitioner's feelings. The widespread use of the model in consultation analysis has in itself gone some way to reducing the denial so prevalent among practitioners about their own emotional needs. In other words, reference to the model legitimizes the recognition and discussion of feelings.

'Here and now awareness' and muscle tone adjustment are two simple stress management techniques which can be easily employed in a consultation. 'Spot the projection' and 'spot the stereotype' go further because they begin the process of analysis of what is happening in a difficult consultation. These are important first steps in identifying why a patient may seem to be rubbing you up the wrong way because they draw attention to the echoes which have been elicited from previous relationships and to the tacit assumptions which each practitioner brings to the consultation. These theme are elaborated by Norton and Smith in a book devoted specifically to the topic of 'problems with patients'.

Problems with patients (Norton and Smith, 1994)

Norton and Smith point out that terms like heartsink represent *stigmatic* labelling. Once such a label is applied, the practitioner's 'capacity for empathy or even sympathy is diminished. In the process the doctor becomes disempowered. By focusing on the stigmatized attributes of patients, their "stupidity" or "hypochondriasis", doctors place their patients out of professional reach because the valid medical task the patients present is relegated in importance, ignored or avoided'. They also note that 'the patient may be blamed for the feelings. When this happens, it is as if the patient is held totally responsible for generating the doctor's discomfort. What began as a professional encounter, with more or less discrete clinical goals, is in danger of becoming little more than a clash of personalities'.

Instead of the term 'heartsink', they propose thinking about 'problems *with* patients' as a way of focusing on the practitioner–patient interaction. In order to provide a 'coherent theoretical framework' and a systematic approach to intervening when there are problems, they combine psychodynamic, social role and systems theories to produce a model which recognizes 'straightforward' and 'complicated' transactions. In order to spot the early warning signs of a complicated transaction, they draw attention to the division between the 'public domain' and the 'personal domain'. In the public domain, practitioners and patients have accepted social roles; sometimes a conflict may become apparent when the practitioner does not elicit the patient's health beliefs but makes false assumptions about them. In the personal domain, the various attributes that make up practitioners and patients as unique individuals are considered, together with the potentially volatile interactions which may result. For example, 'doctors as "givers" for their own personal reasons, may have difficulty when their 'gifts' are not gratefully received by their patients. Patients may experience difficulty in securing help, either because they find it hard to ask for, or have difficulty receiving it or both'.

The psychodynamic perspective is helpful in identifying some individuals who have reality distorting mechanisms which can, for example, lead to an experience of self as fluctuating between extremes of goodness and worthlessness or which might generate enormous anxiety in the face of an authority figure or the breaking of bad news. Awareness of these mechanisms can help the doctor to minimize his own 'bewilderment and frustration'. Conversely, some practitioners may have chosen their careers, largely unconsciously, because of the ability of their public role, status and professional training to compensate for low self-esteem. When patients are submissive, passive and grateful, the practitioner's unconscious needs are being met, but when they are not, the early stages of a complicated clinical transaction are created.

Perhaps the most helpful part of Norton and Smith's work is their systematic approach to interventions which may return a complicated transaction to a straightforward one if the signs are picked up at an early enough stage. They suggest that the main aim is to make explicit any personal issue for either participant which has resulted in departure from the straightforward. By raising such personal matters into the 'public domain', it is hoped that such factors can be openly discussed allowing the doctor and patient to continue their 'collaborative efforts ... conforming to their usual, conventional social roles'. They consider information about the patient which may be helpful to elucidate in four main categories, as shown in Box 14.7.

Box 14.7 Helpful information about patients (Norton and Smith, 1994).

1 Family and wider social network influences.
2 Style and quality of past and current relationships.
3 Personality and level of social functioning.
4 Current relationship with the practitioner and prevailing mood state.

Norton and Smith illustrate these approaches with excellent real examples and use a special analytical technique, called the transaction window, to consider the public and personal aspects of practitioner and patient. For example, Figure 14.3 shows the factors involved in a straightforward clinical transaction.

	Doctor	Patient

Public	(5) Suitably trained
	(7) Able to accurately diagnose
	(8) Able to deliver appropriate
	    treatment/advice/
	    explanation
		(1) Patient seeks appropriate
		    health care
		(2) Has an accurate self-perception
		    of illness and/or symptoms
		(4) Timely presentation to doctor
		(9) Accepts treatment/advice
		    and information
		(10) Returns to acceptable level
		    of health

Personal	(6) Well-disposed toward patient	(3) Trusts doctor

Figure 14.3 Factors involved in a straightforward transaction.

A complicated transaction can be analysed with respect to these 'pre-conditions of the straightforward transaction'. Finding the area in which departure from the straightforward has occurred does not imply anything about the origins of the complication. Norton and Smith give the example of a sensitive patient who is offended at a personal level by the doctor's brusque style and fails to comply with treatment, providing evidence of complication at the public level. These interactions between the public and personal domains are represented by arrows between the cells. The example just described is represented in Figure 14.4.

The authors go on to show how easy it is to use such windows for describing systems, such as the doctor's family, the patient's relatives or aspects of the health service which may be exerting powerful external influences on the consultation.

Critical comments

Norton and Smith have made an extremely valuable contribution in outlining a model of doctor–patient interaction which uses the assumptions underlying the straightforward transaction as a means

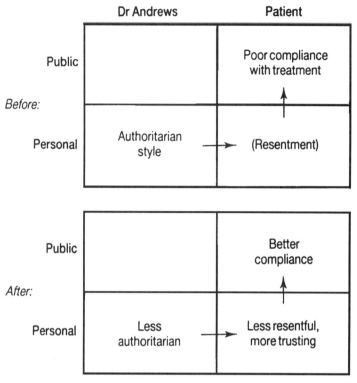

Figure 14.4 An example of a complicated transaction.

of classifying the many types of complication that can arise. The obvious complexity of the practitioner–patient relationship is recognized and yet there is an appealing simplicity to the transaction window approach.

Many readers will not be familiar with the details of psycho-dynamic and systems theories and may be suspicious of terms such as counter-transference and isomorphism which are elaborated in their book.

Some of the patients who cause most unhappiness for practi-tioners have personality disorders and Norton and Smith relegate discussion of this to a short appendix. This may well have been wise because of the complexity of the psychiatric literature on this topic. Linehan provides a detailed analysis of this area and a model of 'dialectical behavioural therapy' which has been extremely influen-tial (Linehan, 1993) but which is not referred to by Norton and Smith.

Despite these reservations, the approach to diagnosis of disturbances within the consultation is more systematic than any other and, most importantly, this helps to generate the most appropriate interventions for 'problems with patients'. In the process the stigmatizing label of 'heartsink' has been effectively exposed, making it significantly harder to speak the word after reading their book. This has to be a good thing.

CONCLUSIONS

The literature on this topic is illuminating because it reflects the human complexity of interactions between practitioners and patients. The categories suggested by Groves do seem to sum up some patients. His insistence that a practitioner's feelings may provide diagnostic information and the importance of examining the goals of care are echoed in nearly all the other papers presented.

Two different approaches to the epidemiology of heartsink concentrated on the patients and the doctors respectively. O'Dowd showed how the label of heartsink may not always be a permanent one and how simple interventions supported by multidisciplinary teamwork appeared effective, at least for some patients. Mathers, on the other hand, showed how the variation between doctors in applying the heartsink label appeared to be related in part to training in communication skills and higher qualifications.

The importance of using colleagues to discuss difficult consultations is emphasized in the 'heartsink survival pack' and helpful strategies for somatizing patients and problem consultations are suggested. Neighbour's concept of housekeeping legitimizes the expression of feelings and he introduces a psychodynamic viewpoint in considering how practitioners may project feelings elicited in previous significant relationships onto patients. Finally, Norton and Smith take psychodynamic explanations further. They describe a framework which is both complex enough to reflect the reality of practitioner–patient interactions and simple enough to provide an accessible tool for analysing the 'complicated' transaction.

Without opportunities for reflection and without the objectivity of a trusted colleague or group, it is easy to use terms like 'heartsink' and to be, sometimes unconsciously, punitive to such patients. The most important message that comes out of the literature is the value of self-awareness. Small group work can be particularly helpful in reflecting on consultations but considerable effort is required to incorporate such an approach into routine practice.

ACTION PLAN

So why did you dip into this chapter? Did any of the descriptions of problems with patients have echoes in your own experience? Reflect for a moment on your starting point. Before going into action planning mode, do some 'housekeeping'. It may be that you want to go to original sources to read more about the ideas summarized here. Or it may be that getting help within the practice or in a small group of peers is more appropriate than reading. If you wish, try our standard checklist to generate your own action plan.

Reflection stop

- Which of your questions remain unanswered?
- Which further sources of information do you feel you need?
- What type of audit might be most helpful?
- What changes have you thought of?
- What resources are available?
- Who else should be involved?

REFERENCES

Adler, G. (1972) Helplessness in the helpers. *British Journal of Medical Psychology*, **45**, 315–326.

Balint, M. (1964) *The Doctor, his Patient and the Illness*, 2nd edn. London: Pitman Medical.

Bowman, F., Goldberg, D., and Millar, T. (1992) Improving the skills of established general practitioners: the long term benefits of group teaching. *Medical Education*, **26**, 63–68.

Ellis, C. (1986) Making dysphoria a happy experience. *British Medical Journal*, **293**, 317–318.

Groves, J. (1978) Taking care of the hateful patient. *New England Journal of Medicine*, **298**, 883–887.

Linehan, M. (1993) *Cognitive-behavioral Treatment of Borderline Personality Disorder*. New York: The Guilford Press.

Mathers, N., and Gask, L. (1995) Surviving the 'heartsink' experience. *Family Practice*, **12**, 176–183.

Mathers, N., Jones, N., and Hannay, D. (1995) Heartsink patients: a study of their general practitioners. *British Journal of General Practice*, **45**, 293–296.

McDonald, P., and O'Dowd, T. (1991) The heartsink patient: a preliminary study. *Family Practice*, **8**, 112–116.

Middleton, J. (1994) Written lists in the consultation: attitudes of general practitioners and the patients who bring them. *British Journal of General Practice*, **44**, 309–310.

Neighbour, R. (1987) *The Inner Consultation*. London: MTP Press.

Norton, K., and Smith, S. (1994) *Problems with Patients: Managing Complicated Transactions*. Cambridge: Cambridge University Press.

O'Dowd, T. (1988) Five years of heartsink patients in general practice. *British Medical Journal*, **297**, 528–530.

Pendleton, D., and Bochner, S. (1980) The communication of medical information in general practice consultations as a function of patients' social class. *Social Sciences and Medicine*, **14A**, 669–673.

15

Cervical screening

WHY IS THIS A HOT TOPIC?

Screening tests have been discussed in some detail in the first section of this book. Cervical screening in the Nordic countries involved nearly complete coverage of the population and was soon followed by a reduction in the total incidence and mortality from carcinoma of the cervix. The past failure of the UK programme seems mainly to have been due to problems with 'organization, accountability and commitment' (Austoker, 1994). Since the 1990 contract, targets for screening have been set and there was an increase in coverage of the target population from 60% to more than 80% within 3 years (Austoker, 1994). General practice has been focusing on this topic.

A critical incident might spur you on to further reading. For example, a patient with an abnormal smear might have become extremely anxious and convinced she has cancer. Alternatively, a patient in whom a recent smear was negative might have developed a symptomatic carcinoma. Or a woman might come in clutching an article from *The Times* entitled 'Is cervical screening really worthwhile? . . . new doubts about smear test' (Drife, 1995).

Cervical screening is a screening test used mainly in the primary care setting where a few papers from the published literature may illuminate the strengths and limitations of this screening programme and help to answer these questions.

Reflection stop

Before reading on, pause and make a list of the main problems with the cervical screening programme as you experience it in your practice. Then compare what you have written with the points we have chosen to highlight in 'Working knowledge' below.

We will be using the 'hot topic framework' and start with 'Working knowledge'.

Box 15.1 Hot topic framework.

1 Working knowledge
2 Individual papers
3 Latest findings
4 Models
5 Action plan

WORKING KNOWLEDGE

A primary health care team pooling their experience of cervical screening would probably highlight some of the following issues.

Screening does seem to pick up some cases of severe *dyskaryosis* which can be referred for effective treatment. If 100 women with CIN are given a smear test, the test will pick up 85 cases of *dyskaryosis*, i.e. 85% sensitivity. If a second smear is performed, this rises to 97%. In primary care, most women who attend have no abnormality and only a few have dyskaryosis. This means that the problems associated with false positive results (and reflected in the specificity of the test) seem to occur more often than the problems of false negatives.

Enormous anxiety can be generated by the results of smear tests, particularly when the 'lab is being cautious'. Inflammatory smears and mild dyskaryosis can be easily misinterpreted by patients as signifying cancer. Effective communication is important both in pre-test counselling and in giving results of such tests to patients.

Some low-risk women seem keen to have annual smears while some of those at higher risk are reluctant to have a smear at all. This may be an example of the 'inverse care law' which implies that greater amounts of care are provided to those who need it least and vice versa (Tudor Hart, 1971). The general concept of targets based on the proportion of the population covered rather than the number of smears performed (item-of-service) certainly seems to make sense in epidemiological terms (Austoker, 1994). To make it work, it is essential to have a good call and recall system (Smith, Elkind and Eardley, 1989).

WHY THESE PAPERS WERE CHOSEN

In this chapter we consider five main areas:

1 The problem of explaining the concept of pre-cancer. We chose a paper from Cardiff (Wilkinson, Jones and McBride, 1990) because it was brief and came up with some very practical suggestions.
2 The natural history of carcinoma of the cervix and the problem of interval cancers which arise suddenly after a truly normal smear. We chose a review article (Wilkinson, 1992) because it summarized clearly current thinking in a journal aimed at GPs. We also chose an audit of deaths which came from a journal aimed at pathologists (Majeed *et al.*, 1994). This retrospective survey looked at factors which seemed to have been important in failing to prevent the condition.
3 Some aspects of organization of the screening programme, in particular consumer orientation, are discussed with reference to a number of papers.
4 Recent research which aims to target women at higher risk of carcinoma for more frequent smears (Wilkinson *et al.*, 1994a). This is a fascinating research area which aims to use knowledge derived from epidemiological studies and translate it into a practical system which might lead to direct patient benefit.
5 The health belief model and how it can explain the woman's perspective when deciding whether or not to go for a smear test. We chose a paper which provides a good introduction to this model (Gillam, 1991) and illustrates the model by what is known about cervical screening.

INDIVIDUAL PAPERS

Now let us consider the ideas and evidence from these papers.

Anxiety caused by abnormal result of cervical smear test (Wilkinson, Jones and McBride, 1990)

Pre-cancer is a difficult concept to explain to patients. This study found significantly less anxiety in patients sent a personalized letter plus a health education leaflet. In a control group receiving the previously used 'standard' letter, 60% assumed they had cancer. The term 'early warning cells' was found to be useful.

Critical comment

This study is important in showing how easy it is for a person to jump to the wrong conclusion when receiving news about a test. Doctors and nurses sometimes forget how it feels to be on the 'receiving end'. Relatively simple interventions (a personalized letter and an information leaflet) led to an improvement. This study also emphasized how important it is to use words which are easily comprehensible. The simple term 'early warning cells' changed the way in which many practitioners gave advice about the results of tests. Not many papers of less than a page long have such a profound effect on clinical practice. Perhaps this is an example of the SAS (short and simple) principle, which is said to be a key ingredient for success in audit.

Abnormal cervical smear test results: old dilemmas and new directions (Wilkinson, 1992)

This helpful review article summarizes current thinking on natural history. The author points out that there has been a great increase in CIN1 in the last few decades but little change in the prevalence of CIN3. If all patients with CIN1 were immediately referred to hospital, colposcopy clinics would be swamped. There is general agreement that CIN2 and 3 should be treated. If CIN1 persists for 6 months, referral is probably indicated. The natural history of cervical dysplasia is poorly understood: most cases of CIN1 regress rather than progressing. The concept is emerging that dysplasia is a dichotomy not a continuum. This may also help explain interval cancers arising after a truly normal smear.

Critical comment

One of the criteria for successful screening is that the natural history of the condition should be well understood; there remain many unanswered questions for carcinoma of the cervix. The most obvious is how true interval cancers arise *de novo* without prior dysplastic changes.

Using patient and general practice characteristics to explain variations in cervical smear uptake rates (Majeed et al., 1994)

This was a retrospective audit of 36 deaths from carcinoma of the cervix over 2 years. The authors looked at primary care and hospital notes and reviewed smears. They noted that 40% of deaths were in those over 65 years and emphasized the importance of offering smear tests to women of this age if they had no previous smear. Four main factors were identified which seemed roughly equal in importance:

1 Women not invited.
2 Invited but did not attend.
3 True negative recent smear, i.e. interval cancer.
4 False negative smear.

Interval cancers could be minimized by reducing the screening interval to 3 years in all districts. The fact that a few interval cancers occur means that no screening programme can hope to prevent cervical cancer completely. This is clearly a limitation when compared with the criteria for effective screening.

The authors suggest that false negative smears could be minimized by introducing a 'rapid screening technique' for quality assurance within laboratories with a 30-second scan by an independent cytologist. This has been shown to be more effective than re-analysing a random 10% sample of smears.

Critical comment

Although this was simply an audit looking back at case notes, it was helpful in highlighting the fact that carcinoma of the cervix is predominantly a disease of the older woman. It is difficult to eliminate bias in retrospective studies, so it may be hard to judge the relative contribution of the factors identified as important in failing to make the diagnosis for these women. Nevertheless, it is helpful to have a succinct list of the problem areas. Because this audit was initiated by pathologists, the implications for quality control within the laboratory are discussed. The details of this are not of direct relevance to primary care practitioners, but some knowledge of quality control may be helpful in answering questions from women about what happens to the smear test slide after it leaves the surgery.

Consumer orientation of screening

Making cervical screening work (Smith, Elkind and Eardley, 1989)

This review article emphasizes that complete population coverage is the ideal and discusses some of the problems which have prevented this, such as the inadequacy of computerized databases, particularly in urban areas. The provision of the service should be convenient and acceptable to women. The jargon used to describe this is: consumer oriented but service initiated (COSI). An example of consumer orientation is described in another paper (Chomet and Chomet, 1990). An invitation with a specific appointment is sent to coincide with a woman's birthday and the birthday gift offered is a cervical smear test!

Can health education increase uptake of cervical smear testing among Asian women? (McAvoy and Raza, 1991)

Asian women who had never had a smear were contacted and different types of health education material compared: written material sent by post, personal visit with a leaflet, personal visit with a video. Eleven percent of those sent leaflets had a smear in the next 4 months compared with 37% visited and given a leaflet and 47% of those visited and shown a video.

Critical comment

These papers emphasize the importance of making the screening programme accessible and acceptable to women. Health education interventions do need to be tested so that cost-effectiveness can be determined. The study from Leicester, targeting Asian women, is a good example of targeting a specific group and comparing different interventions.

LATEST FINDINGS

An important research project has been reported in a number of papers. The authors used epidemiologically known 'risk factors' to derive an index of increased risk and have reported preliminary findings of applying this in primary care.

Risk targeting in cervical screening (Wilkinson et al., 1994a, 1994b)

A simple scoring system has been derived from a survey of studies of risk factors for CIN and carcinoma of cervix. Four main risk factors were identified: number of sexual partners; years of use of the oral contraceptive pill; current smoking status; and absence of higher education. This scoring system could be used not to deny smears to low-risk women but perhaps to increase the frequency of testing offered to higher-risk women. Studies showed score results were highly repeatable when test–retest comparisons were made and that self-reporting was acceptable to women despite the 'highly personal' questions asked. Those with high scores were at higher risk of CIN than those with low scores: the former group were labelled the 'low-risk group' and the latter the 'very low-risk group' to reduce the anxiety provoking impact of a label such as 'higher risk'. The former group (20% of a large sample) had an 11-fold increase in rates of CIN2 and 3 in a prospective study and this accounted for 75% of all the histologically proven cases.

Critical comment

Many will be aware of the epidemiological risk factors associated with higher prevalence of cervical dyskaryosis, but the work applying this theoretical knowledge in the form of risk group targeting is less widely known. The potential looks promising. However, critical appraisal must mention the need for careful evaluation of effectiveness and workload implications before widespread adoption of such an approach in practice. This is where the skills developed in the first section of the book can be most helpful; in asking questions about generalizability and consequences of results from a specific research paper.

MODELS

The patient's perspective is obviously important when one asks why some women have smear tests and others do not. A number of potential deterrents to being screened have been identified (Box 15.2) and a helpful model (the Health Belief Model) has been applied.

Box 15.2 Deterrents to having a smear test.

- Failure to receive invitation.
- Ignorance of test (e.g. 'it's only for the promiscuous').
- Fear of disease (e.g. 'it's a cancer test').
- Lack of female staff/embarrassment/discomfort.
- Misconceptions about disease ('no need once you're past the change').
- Inconvenient time or location of testing.
- Unhappy past experience of having a test.

Gillam (Gillam, 1991) has pointed out that the Health Belief Model is helpful in considering such deterrents. The model has four key concepts (Box 15.3).

Box 15.3 Key concepts of the health belief model.

1 Behaviour of individuals is essentially rational.
2 Behaviour is understandable only in terms of beliefs.
3 Understanding is required before a **belief** can be modified.
4 This is the first step in modification of **behaviour**.

When assessing health beliefs, the model includes five elements (Box 15.4).

Box 15.4 Five elements of health beliefs.

1 Motivation.
2 Perceived vulnerability.
3 Perceived seriousness.
4 Perceived cost/benefit.
5 Cues to action.

Gillam applies this model to the uptake of cervical screening (Gillam, 1991). A summary of his main points follows:

- **Motivation**:   Difficult to measure.

  High uptake of screening in upper social classes.

  This is likely to be due to more than just differences in 'motivation'.

- **Vulnerability**:   Some women believe falsely that:

  'there's little risk after menopause' or

  'it's only for the promiscuous'.

- **Seriousness**:   Seriousness not doubted but balanced by fear

  Anxiety increased by: delay in getting results, and by technical terms, e.g. 'CIN'

- **Cost/benefit**:   Pain and embarrassment of major concern; access to a woman doctor important

  Time and cost of attending (?related social class)

- **Cues to action**:   Many attend without invitation; this has been little studied. Some women learn of the test from their grand-daughters.

Critical comments

In applying a screening test in primary care, the majority receiving the test will be healthy individuals who are not affected by the condition being sought. For this reason, it is particularly important to 'do no harm' and a formalized consideration of the woman's point of view is extremely helpful. It is particularly important to obtain informed consent before performing a test which to the practitioner may be routine but which to the woman may represent a serious personal invasion: coercion must be avoided.

A crucial factor for success is coverage of the target population and this model provides a framework for considering the factors which need to be addressed in making a screening programme user-friendly. The style, tone, presentation and contents of the letter of invitation are very important. A review article (Austoker, 1994) emphasizes that those most at risk are older women from lower social classes. In organizing screening, achieving a wide coverage of ages is a more important determinant of risk reduction than the frequency of screening. For this reason, health professionals may need to focus attention on the ageist false belief which has been highlighted: 'there's no need to bother once you're past the menopause'.

MAIN CONCEPTS REVIEWED

When considering how closely cervical smear testing fits the criteria for a screening programme, a number of important points emerge, some very practical, such as the problems associated with obtaining accurate population registers and operating effective call and recall, and some to do with the natural history of the disease. The problem of interval cancers has been discussed as well as the dichotomous model of cytological abnormalities (CIN1 and 2 versus CIN3 and 4). Psychological aspects of screening must be taken into account and the term 'early warning cells' is useful in explaining dyskaryosis to patients. It is helpful to take a patient-centred approach in considering deterrents to being screened as this may suggest ways of improving uptake of screening and the health belief model provides a useful framework. Finally, the work on targeting women with higher risk may offer benefits once the effectiveness and implications of this approach have been widely tested.

LESSONS WHICH MAY APPLY TO OTHER TOPICS

Note that the focus on psychological aspects of screening and deterrents to being screened was based on our 'working knowledge' of the problems associated with cervical smear tests. This emphasizes the importance of using such knowledge as a starting point in selecting what to read. There is a fascinating literature on the psychological aspects of screening (Marteau, 1989).

You do not need to read many long and complicated articles: very often the shortest will be the best. The shortest article referred to in this chapter is less than a page long but contains the simple but powerful explanation of 'early warning cells'. This concept can be incorporated with immediate benefit into clinical practice without the need for randomized controlled trials!

ACTION PLAN

At the beginning of this chapter, we suggested that you make a list of the main problems with the cervical screening programme as you experience it in your own practice. How similar and how different were your areas of concern to those we have chosen to highlight? Before making an action plan, reflect a little on whether any more information is needed.

Reflection stop

- Which of your questions remain unanswered?
- Which further sources of information do you feel you need?
- What type of audit might be most helpful?
- What changes have you thought of?
- What resources are available?
- Who else should be involved?

REFERENCES

Austoker, J. (1994) Screening for cervical cancer. *British Medical Journal*, **309**, 241–247.

Chomet, J., and Chomet, J. (1990) Cervical screening in general practice: a 'new' scenario. *British Medical Journal*, **300**, 1504–1506.

Drife, J. (1995) Is cervical screening really worthwhile? *The Times*, 17–10–95 Times Newspapers Ltd.

Gillam, S.J. (1991) Understanding the uptake of cervical cancer screening: the contribution of the health belief model. [Review]. *British Journal of General Practice*, **41**, 510–513.

Majeed, F.A., Cook, D.G., Anderson, H.R., Hilton, S., Bunn, S., and Stones, C. (1994) Using patient and general practice characteristics to explain variations in cervical smear uptake rates. *British Medical Journal*, **308**, 1272–1276.

Marteau, T. (1989) Psychological costs of screening. *British Medical Journal*, **299**, 527.

McAvoy, B.R., and Raza, R. (1991) Can health education increase uptake of cervical smear testing among Asian women? *British Medical Journal*, **302**, 833–836.

Smith, A., Elkind, A., and Eardley, A. (1989) Making cervical screening work. *British Medical Journal*, **298**, 1662–1664.

Tudor Hart, J. (1971) The inverse care law. *Lancet*, **1**, 405–412.

Wilkinson, C. (1992) Abnormal cervical smear test results: old dilemmas and new directions. *British Journal of General Practice*, **42**, 336–339.

Wilkinson, C., Jones, J.M., and McBride, J. (1990) Anxiety caused by abnormal result of cervical smear test: a controlled trial. *British Medical Journal*, **300**, 440.

Wilkinson, C.E., Peters, T.J., Harvey, I.M., and Stott, N.C. (1994a) Feasibility, reliability and women's views of a risk scoring system for cervical neoplasia in primary care. *British Journal of General Practice*, **44**, 306–308.

Wilkinson, C.E., Peters, T.J., Stott, N.C., and Harvey, I.M. (1994b) Prospective evaluation of a risk scoring system for cervical neoplasia in primary care. *British Journal of General Practice*, **44**, 341–344.

16

Referrals to outpatient clinics

WHY IS THIS A HOT TOPIC?

We are working within a managed health service where rationing decisions are increasingly explicit. The aim is for a primary care-led NHS and general practice has always fulfilled a gatekeeper role in making referrals to secondary care. Since the 1990 contract, there has been a requirement for general practitioners to include details of referrals, broken down by speciality, in an annual report. This change in Terms and Conditions of Service followed a recognition of the wide variations in referral rates as well as a frustration felt by many in the Department of Health that such variations were largely unexplained (Wilkin, 1992). A number of levels have been described (Box 16.1).

Box 16.1 Three levels of variation in referral rate.

1 Between districts.
2 Between practitioners working within the same district.
3 Between practitioners working within the same practice.

Such variation inevitably raises questions about whether high-referring doctors are wasting resources by making inappropriate referrals or whether low-referring doctors are denying their patients access to treatments which might be beneficial.

In this chapter, we will again use the hot topic framework.

Box 16.2 Hot topic framework.

1 Working knowledge
2 Individual papers
3 Latest findings
4 Models
5 Action plan

WORKING KNOWLEDGE

There appears to be a significant tension between looking at referrals in profession-led and service-led ways which depends partly on the purpose of the exercise. An example of a profession-led approach would be peer review looking at individual referrals with the purpose of educating the practitioner and improving knowledge and awareness of criteria for appropriate referral. An example of a service-led approach might be a health authority initiative where the main purpose was seen by practices as being downward pressure on costs (e.g. guidelines on referral which are perceived as being 'imposed'). This would understandably be treated with suspicion by doctors who are concerned to protect their clinical freedom as gatekeepers of the NHS.

The importance of the GP's gatekeeper role has been further emphasized with the development of the purchaser–provider split which has stimulated a greater awareness of decisions about purchasing secondary care and about the factors influencing the referral process. Of course, service and professional agendas are not mutually exclusive and the increasing interest in evidence-based medicine may help to reconcile what appear to be different viewpoints.

One of the critical incidents which might lead you to read the literature on referrals might be a practice visit from a member of the Health Authority who has costs at the top of his agenda. Alternatively, you might yourself be involved in commissioning decisions on behalf of your practice or within your locality. Either way a brief look at the evidence on the process of hospital referrals will reveal a complex but fascinating subject which offers insights but no easy answers.

WHY THE PAPERS WERE CHOSEN

In this chapter we will choose five areas to consider:

1 Explaining variation in referral rates.
2 The role of clinical uncertainty in referral.
3 Knowledge of a speciality and referral to that speciality.
4 Attempts to alter referral patterns.
5 Models of the referral process.

Two key review articles, which are widely quoted, make a starting point in considering the factors which may explain variation in referral (Wilkin, 1992; Wilkin and Smith, 1987). A good piece of qualitative research (Newton *et al.*, 1991) used interview techniques to assess GP's motivation in making referrals and highlighted many important non-clinical factors.

The role of clinical uncertainty was highlighted in a study from Oxford which also looked at variations in both referral rate and in admission rate following a referral to outpatients (Coulter *et al.*, 1990).

Knowledge of a speciality may increase referrals in that speciality and a simple general practice audit provides some evidence for this (Reynolds *et al.*, 1991).

There have been several papers describing either attempts to alter referral patterns (usually unsuccessful) or considering whether guidelines on referral would be helpful in reducing the referral rate. Three papers will be discussed (de Marco *et al.*, 1993; Fertig *et al.*, 1993; McColl *et al.*, 1994) under the heading 'Latest findings'.

Under 'models', we will look at an article which provides evidence of the importance of patient expectation (Webb and Lloyd,

1994) and then we will conclude by looking briefly at one of the attempts which have been made to map the cognitive processes involved in the decision to refer (Jones, 1992).

Pause for a moment and consider the questions in the Reflection stop box.

Reflection stop

Before reading on answer two brief questions:

1 How would you measure your own referral rate?
2 Write a short list of factors which you think might influence the referral rate, perhaps using 'Doctor factors', 'Practice and secondary care factors' and 'Patient factors' as headings. A list of factors which others have postulated as potentially important is given below.

CALCULATING YOUR OWN REFERRAL RATE

Referral rates may be measured and expressed in a number of different ways and a helpful review summarizes this area (Roland, 1992). Keeping copies of typed referral letters is the simplest method of finding the number of referrals but those made by telephone, hand-written letter or by deputies and locums may be missed. Monitoring incoming letters from hospitals may provide additional information if records are reviewed of patients where the referral has not already been noted, but this can be time-consuming. Computerized systems are popular but the quality of data obviously depends on the continuing motivation of users. A final problem is whether to include or exclude private referrals from the analysis.

The bigger problem is how to express the number of referrals as a rate. Should the denominator be list size, number of consultations or number of patients seen? For comparing practices, the number of referrals per 1000 patients per year is often used; in other words dividing the total number of referrals by the total number of patients. But practice rates are unlikely to be a useful basis for self-audit and voluntary peer review or for discussion between the Health Authority and an individual GP (Roland *et al.*, 1990). Here the individual list size should not be used as it takes no account of major differences in workload and using the number of consultations carried out by a doctor is better.

Factors which might influence referral rate are:

- **Doctor factors**
  Age and sex
  Experience of a speciality
  Training and qualifications
  Use of investigations
  Case-mix of patients usually seen
  Unexplained variation from one time to another
- **Practice and secondary care factors**
  List size
  Number of ancillary staff
  Number of partners
  Intra-practice referrals
  Workload patterns, e.g. consultation rate
  Geographical location
  Distance to nearest hospital
  Availability of transport
  Range and availability of hospital services
- **Patient factors**
  Social class
  Age and sex
  Morbidity and health care 'need'
  Deprivation index of area
  Patient expectation

This list is certainly not comprehensive and you will probably have identified other factors which might influence referral rates.

INDIVIDUAL PAPERS

Now let us turn to some individual papers. First we will see what the literature has to say about some of the factors mentioned above.

1 Explaining variation in referral rates

The evidence has been carefully reviewed in two important papers (Wilkin, 1992; Wilkin and Smith, 1987). To summarize a large research area, it would be fair to say that there is no clear evidence for any of these factors alone having a major influence on explaining differences in referral rate. 'It should not be surprising to find that a complex problem does not yield easily to crude and simple methods' (Wilkin and Smith, 1987). 'The selection of independent variables has largely been based on what was readily available or easily collected rather than on what might be considered theoretically most important' (Wilkin, 1992).

Interpreting differences in referral rates is fraught with hazard as rates are often derived from short studies and there appear to be huge variations simply due to random variation. A doctor may find himself a high referrer one month but a low referrer the next. There is even more scope for sampling error if rates are looked at by speciality. Such errors probably contribute highly to those studies which report 20-fold variation in referral rates. Studies over longer periods often yield variation in rates of 2–4-fold (Moore and Roland, 1989; Wilkin, 1992).

One of the factors generally ignored from analysis of crude rates is the purpose of the referral (Wilkin and Smith, 1987). Box 16.3 summarizes some of these.

Box 16.3 Simple classification of purpose of referral (Wilkin and Smith, 1987).

- For diagnosis
- For investigation
- For treatment
- For advice
- For a combination of these
- At patient insistence

Critical comment

Once one asks about the reasons for referrals, the whole process of the consultation suddenly becomes relevant as the background against which the decision to refer is made. For the moment all one can say is that most of the variation among doctors in referral rates is unexplained. Some restate this as 'the greatest variable is the doctor' or invoke the concept of different 'referral thresholds' (Cummins *et al.*, 1981) without actually being able to provide evidence of the reasons for the differences.

Northumberland study (Newton et al., 1991)

This was a small qualitative survey based on interviews with 15 GPs. It involved discussion of three recent individual referrals for 1 hour with a follow-up interview. This type of approach concerns itself with **perceptions, meanings** and **motives** and the authors contrast it with the 'positivist approach' which looks at high and low referrers and tries to identify easily measurable differences (e.g. sex, qualifications etc) usually with little success in explaining differences.

The study emphasized the complexity of interacting factors leading to a referral decision and found that referral often occurred after several consultations and that social, cultural and non-clinical factors were important. Some of the non-clinical doctor factors identified are summarized in Box 16.4.

Box 16.4 Non-clinical doctor factors affecting the decision to refer (Newton *et al.*, 1991).

- Willingness to tolerate uncertainty.
- Concern over medico-legal aspects.
- Concern over relationship of GP to consultant.
- Attitude of GP to patient's right to second opinion.
- Relationship with partners: intra-practice referral.
- Referral as means of education or testing the service.
- Doctor's personal values and concepts of care.

The authors concluded that a large number of referral decisions are difficult to justify on clinical grounds alone. Such decisions are clearly complicated by personal values, skills and experiences of those involved and especially by the relationships between GP, patient, partners and consultants. These factors were summarized as 'the environment of decision making'.

Critical comment

The term 'the environment of decision making' does not in itself explain anything but it does summarize nicely the complexities of referral. The richness of factors involved and the sheer humanity of the process are well illustrated by this paper.

The role of clinical uncertainty in referral

Relation between general practices' outpatient referral rates and rates of elective admission to hospital' (Coulter et al., 1990)

This Oxford based study looked at the relationship between outpatient referral rates and subsequent elective admission rates. Overall, most practices with high referral rates also had high admission rates. If these practices had been referring unnecessarily, one might have expected consultants to admit a lower proportion of such patients. The authors concluded that for some specialities at least, practices with average or low rates may be depriving their patients of beneficial hospital treatment. This is an important conclusion since the political agenda sometimes implies that the high-referring doctor or practice is the culprit for wasting resources.

The authors also highlighted uncertainty as a major potential factor in explaining variation in referral rates. Variation was found to be most for specialities where there was most uncertainty about the best investigation and treatment. Overall, admission rates were just as variable as referral rates, 'underlining the uncertainty that characterizes clinical decision making in hospital specialities as well as in general practice'. Finally, the authors concluded that consultants may not be a 'gold standard judge of quality' and that crude referral rates cannot be used to judge quality.

Knowledge of a speciality and referral to that speciality

General practitioner outpatient referrals: do good doctors refer more patients to hospital? (Reynolds et al., 1991)

The provocative title of this article is probably intended to counteract the assumption that high-referring doctors waste resources.

A five-partner training practice with an average overall referral rate analysed about 400 referrals according to speciality. Significant differences were noted between partners in referral rates, particularly for ophthalmology, ENT and dermatology. High rates of referral to a speciality were associated with a doctor having a 'special interest' in the subject. As this could possibly have been due to intra-practice referral of patients or to self-selection of patients attending a particular doctor, an analysis of case-mix was performed for a 6-week period. The partner who was a hospital practitioner in ENT made half of the ENT referrals of the practice but only saw a quarter of ENT cases. On the other hand, the partner making 81% of eye referrals saw 57% of eye cases in the practice, so case mix selection may have contributed to the high rate in this case. The high rate was not due to lack of confidence in that speciality, as the 'special interest' of the doctor was reported as associated with 'feeling more confident than average' in managing conditions within that speciality.

The authors concluded that a high referral rate does not necessarily indicate inappropriate referral.

Critical comment

This was an audit rather than a prospective study, so the results must be treated cautiously. However, the process of analysing the referrals from a practice retrospectively could be done in most practices without creating the sometimes artificial circumstances of a prospective study. This is what gives the results their appeal. The contrast between ENT and ophthalmology referrals serves to underline the fact that sometimes case-mix may cause apparent bias when comparing individual practitioners with each other. The fact that GPs 'with an interest' had high levels of referral to that speciality and did not seem to be referring through lack of confidence is important. It may be that such referrals are generated because of knowledge of what can be done and this would support the authors' conclusions that high levels are not inappropriate. However, there are many other possible explanations which are not explored by this study and which might not suggest quite such appropriateness. For example, it might be that the GP plays golf with the hospital consultant for whom he is clinical assistant and is motivated to refer for reasons which have more to do with that relationship than to do with specific aspects of patient care. This is an extreme example of 'the environment of decision making' already discussed.

LATEST FINDINGS

Attempts to alter referral patterns

How valuable is feedback of information on hospital referral patterns? (de Marco et al., 1993)

Audit facilitators visited surgeries to discuss referral rates. Most GPs were naturally defensive, were unenthusiastic about using information provided for audit and were sceptical about the accuracy of the data. GP's perceptions of the causes of varying referral rates included four main factors which are summarized in Box 16.5.

Box 16.5 GP's perceptions of causes of variation in referral rate (de Marco *et al.*, 1993).

- Access to specialist care/waiting times etc.
- Individual skills of GP.
- Patient expectation and demand.
- Fear of litigation.

The facilitators reported their view that overall rates have no relation to quality of care and form a 'sterile basis for discussion'. They suggested that analysis of individual cases might be better. However, an accompanying editorial written by a professor of Public Health Medicine (Hutchinson, 1993) points out that rejecting analysis of referral rates is 'unsustainable . . . GPs have to accept that information on referrals has a part to play in the effective use of resources'. This is yet another example of the tension between professional and service agendas referred to at the beginning of this chapter.

Understanding variation in rates among general practitioners: are inappropriate referrals important and would guidelines help to reduce rates? (Fertig et al., 1993)

Six hundred referrals were assessed by consultants (100 in each of six specialities). About 10% were judged 'possibly or definitely inappropriate'. A similar proportion were judged by an independent GP not to have followed locally developed guidelines for referral. However, even if these were eliminated, there would still be a wide variation in referral rate, indicating that inappropriate referrals only account for a small part of such variation.

The study concluded that the introduction of guidelines would be unlikely to alter the number of referrals made: if guidelines are adhered to strictly, a few patients would be referred who would not otherwise have been referred as well as a few 'inappropriate referrals' being avoided. This may or may not be a good thing: the main point is that using guidelines in the hope of cutting costs is naïve.

An agenda for change in referral – consensus from general practice (McColl et al., 1994)

The authors of this paper started by recognizing that there is an incomplete understanding of the sources of variation in GP referral rates but pointed out that even in the absence of such understanding, strategies for maximizing benefit from hospital services need to be considered. GPs have a strong sense of professional autonomy and for any change to succeed, those responsible for making it should be involved in setting the agenda. '. . . General practitioners seemed to speak with one voice. They regarded referrals as their business and any initiative designed to change the volume, timing or destination . . . would be commonly regarded as interference.'

The authors therefore sought to find out what GP's priorities were by using the *Delphi technique*, with a series of questionnaires followed up by in-depth qualitative interviews. They found close agreement among GPs irrespective of whether they were high or low referrers, fundholders, in a training practice or whether in rural or urban practice. The priorities for change were formulated by taking into account both the 'amenability to change' of different factors and the 'keenness' with which GPs felt such change should take place, nicely blending motivation with realism. Five main areas were identified (Box 16.7).

Box 16.6 High priority areas for change (McColl *et al.*, 1994).

1 Length of hospital waiting lists.
2 Range of 'open access' services.
3 Medical knowledge and training of GPs.
4 Information about availability of hospital services.
5 Knowledge of and relationship with consultants.

Interest was expressed in a number of initiatives including development of directories of hospital services, structured programmes of continuing education including 'sitting in' on consultant-led clinics and the developments of guidelines for referral including when to use the term 'urgent'.

The authors identified some barriers to change and these are summarized in Box 16.7.

Box 16.7 Six barriers to change (McColl *et al.*, 1994).

1 GP's sense of professional autonomy.
2 Lack of resources.
3 Lack of time.
4 General inertia.
5 Espoused norm of equality: lack of leadership for change.
6 Interprofessional rivalry between GPs and consultants.

Despite these barriers, the researchers point out that the identification of professional priorities is a necessary first step. Meetings between consultants and GPs could then follow to review and improve current referral practice.

Critical comment

It does seem unlikely that the approach suggested in this paper would reduce the costs of health care but it certainly has the potential to improve the quality of care provided. Whether this would be enough to satisfy the demands of 'the service' is largely a political question.

MODELS

Patients' expectations about referral (Webb and Lloyd, 1994)

This study used self-reporting questionnaires, completed in the waiting room, to record each patient's presenting problem and duration as well as the amount of functional limitation and associated anxiety. In addition, patient expectation of the forthcoming consultation was assessed, including whether or not they expected referral. Each of 12 doctors in the study filled in a brief encounter form after the consultation recording patient details, main complaint, diagnosis and action taken. The two sets of data were then matched where possible (about 50% of the forms).

The nature of the presenting problem and functional limitation were both related to patients' expectation about referral. Anxiety was also a significant factor: those with 'considerable or moderate anxiety' were three times more likely to expect referral than those with slight or no anxiety. When it came to matching patient expectation with action taken by GPs, patients who expected a referral were six times more likely to be referred than those who did not. But anxiety itself was not independently associated with an increased likelihood of referral.

Critical comments

The authors point out two possible interpretations. Patient expectation may be based on previous experience and may therefore be quite accurate in predicting doctors' actions. Alternatively patients may be expressing their expectations clearly in the consultation so influencing doctors' behaviour.

Either way, patient expectation is clearly linked to the outcome of the consultation, confirming the hunch expressed in 'Working Knowledge'.

Decision making and hospital referrals (Jones, 1992)

In this useful chapter, Jones describes several models which attempt to perform 'cognitive mapping' of the thoughts which are in operation during the decision-making part of a consultation. Some of these have been derived from a method which uses video stimulated recall, although Jones points out that a practitioner may give an account not of what they actually did or thought but rather of how they thought the problem *should* have been solved. Despite such reservations, some important insights emerge from this approach.

1 Several hypotheses are generated early in a clinical encounter and this is followed by a search for information which will help reject or confirm them.

2 Pattern recognition is important in making a diagnosis. Each individual has a unique and complex knowledge base and there may be variation between clinicians in the key aspects of a patient's history which trigger access to longer term memories. These have been called 'forceful features' (Gale and Marsden, quoted by Jones, 1992).

3 The emotional context of the consultation is important and this may be linked to previous knowledge of the patient.

4 Esteem is a major factor; concern about loss of esteem in the eyes of a consultant, due to an unnecessary referral, has to be balanced against the loss of esteem in the eyes of the patient associated with a missed diagnosis. Clinicians do not like to appear foolish.

5 There are large differences in the degree to which practitioners can tolerate diagnostic uncertainty.

6 There are many reasons for referral other than diagnosis; the likelihood of obtaining 'appropriate management' through referral is also important. So access to coronary angiography may vary according to how keen the local cardiologist is on tertiary referral for surgical intervention.

One of the models quoted by Jones is a framework for looking at the different influences on the referral decision. It comes from a book which highlights the importance of the professional relationship between consultants and GPs (Dowie, 1983). The framework is shown in Figure 16.1.

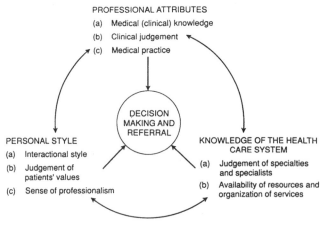

Figure 16.1 Decision making and referral

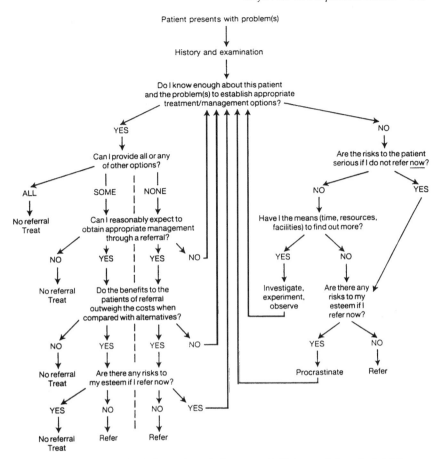

Figure 16.2 A model of the referral decision Wilkin and Smith (1987) reproduced in Jones (1992)

Some have gone further than this framework in trying to map the complex decision-making process. An example is shown in Figure 16.2.

Critical comments

Separating the components involved in decision-making seems a logical thing to do, but sometimes the decision-making 'trees' which result seem mechanistic and counter-intuitive. Do practitioners really go through these questions in a logical step-by-step way? And even if they occasionally do, how do such models help to explain variation? Jones suggests that they are an improvement on models which simply postulate different referral thresholds. He also points out that they 'embrace many factors which fall outside the 'rational' model of medical behaviour'. Beyond this, it is unclear how one could generate testable predictions or new ideas for research. How common is it for a practitioner to be consciously aware of such cognitive processes and do they vary their approach in different contexts, perhaps depending on the degree of perceived risk? Considerable effort appears to have been expended in drawing such maps, but in the process major emotional events, such as anxiety in doctor or patient, have been reduced to rather bland questions such as 'Have I the means to find out more?'. The whole question of usefulness hinges on the purpose to which the model will be put. A major priority, identified by Jones, is to find non-threatening ways of using peer review to improve the referral process, including the communication skills involved in the consultation. Perhaps more research effort should go into looking at this than into finding more and more complex ways of arranging questions and arrows.

MAIN CONCEPTS REVIEWED

There are wide variations in referral rates between doctors and the most obvious and easily measured doctor, patient and health system variables seem to explain only a small part of this variation. The effect of random variation seems to be as big as any of the other factors identified. This must be a frustrating realization for those looking for an easy way to cut health care costs because complex systems subject to multiple small influences are the most difficult to change. It is clear that crude referral rates cannot be used as a measure of quality of care.

Although general practitioners are keen to preserve their independence as 'gatekeepers of the NHS' and resent any suggestions which might curtail that freedom, they have been shown to have their own agenda for improving the process of referral. This is more about improving quality of care than about containing costs. A recent study of referrals from fundholding practices supports this view (Surender et al. 1995). Even without a clear understanding of the factors which influence referral rates, several practical suggestions have been made which will facilitate this process, such as joint locality-based meetings between GPs and consultants for audit, education and the development of guidelines on referral. The link between education and commissioning of care will need to be addressed by Primary Care Groups.

Some of the influences on referral rates are clear from our working knowledge, but others (such as the ability to tolerate diagnostic uncertainty, the real clinical uncertainty which underlies management in some specialities and the importance of esteem in the relationship between practitioners and consultants) are less obvious. The value of qualitative research is highlighted by the crucial insights which this approach has provided. Patient expectation is perceived by doctors as being an important determinant of the decision to refer and this impression has evidence to support it.

The literature also includes models which help our understanding of the cognitive processes involved in making a referral decision. These are beginning to reflect the complexity which one would expect of a decision which is a part of the consultation, with all the personal, ethical and emotional influences which affect the doctor–patient relationship. Further insights will depend on whether such subtle and complex factors can be teased apart so that useful generalizations can be made.

ACTION PLAN

At the beginning of this chapter we asked you to identify your own issues related to the referral process within your own practice. Reflect again on these; they may be very different from the examples we have chosen to discuss in this chapter. Consider what else you need to know before taking action (see Reflection stop box).

Reflection stop

- Which of your questions remain unanswered?
- Which further sources of information do you feel you need?
- What type of audit of asthma care might be most helpful?
- What changes have you thought of?
- What resources are available?
- Who else should be involved?

REFERENCES

Coulter, A., Seagroatt, V., and McPherson, K. (1990) Relation between general practices' outpatient referral rate and rates of elective admission to hospital. *British Medical Journal*, **301**, 273–276.

Cummins, R., Jarman, B., and White, P. (1981) Do general practitioners have different 'referral thresholds'? *British Medical Journal*, **282**, 1037–1039.

de Marco, P., Dain, C., Lockwood, T., and Roland, M. (1993) How valuable is feedback of information on hospital referral patterns? *British Medical Journal*, **307**, 1465–1466.

Dowie, R. (1983) *General practitioners and consultants: a study of outpatient referrals*. London: King's Fund.

Fertig, A., Roland, M., King, H., and Moore, T. (1993)Understanding variation in rates of referral among general practitioners: are inappropriate referrals important and would guidelines help to reduce rates? *British Medical Journal*, **307**, 1467–1470.

Hutchinson, A. (1993) Explaining referral variation. *British Medical Journal*, **307**, 1439

Jones, R. (1992) Decision making and hospital referrals. In: Roland, M. and Coulter, A. (eds.) *Hospital referrals*, pp. 92–106. Oxford: Oxford University Press.

McColl, E., Newton, J. and Hutchinson, A. (1994) An agenda for change in referral – consensus from general practice. *British Journal of General Practice*, **44**, 157–162.

Moore, A., and Roland, M. (1989) How much variation in referral rates among general practitioners is due to chance? *British Medical Journal*, **298**, 500–502.

Newton, J., Hayes, V., and Hutchinson, A. (1991) Factors influencing general practitioners' referral decisions. *Family Practice*, **8**, 308–313.

Reynolds, G., Chitnis, J., and Roland, M. (1991) General practitioner outpatient referrals: do good doctors refer more patients to hospital? *British Medical Journal*, **302**, 1250–1252.

Roland, M., Bartholomew, J., Morrell, D., McDermott, A., and Paul,E. (1990) Understanding hospital referral rates: a user's guide. *British Medical Journal*, **301**, 98–102.

Roland, M. (1992) Measuring referral rates. In: Roland, M. and Coulter, A. (eds.) *Hospital referrals*, pp. 62–75. Oxford: Oxford University Press.

Surender, R., Bradlow, J., Coulter, A., Doll, H., and Stewart Brown, S. (1995) Prospective study of trends in referral patterns in fundholding and non-fundholding practices in the Oxford region, 1990–4. *British Medical Journal*, **311**, 1205–1208.

Webb, S., and Lloyd, M. (1994) Prescribing and referral in general practice: a study of patients' expectation and doctors' actions. *British Journal of General Practice*, **44**, 165–169.

Wilkin, D. (1992) Patterns of referral: explaining variation. In: Roland, M., and Coulter, A. (eds.) *Hospital referrals*, pp. 76–91. Oxford: Oxford University Press.

Wilkin, D., and Smith, A. (1987) Explaining variation in general practitioner referrals to hospital. *Family Practice*, **4**, 160–169.

Index